Psychology of Health - Biopsychosocial Approach

Edited by Simon George Taukeni

Published in London, United Kingdom

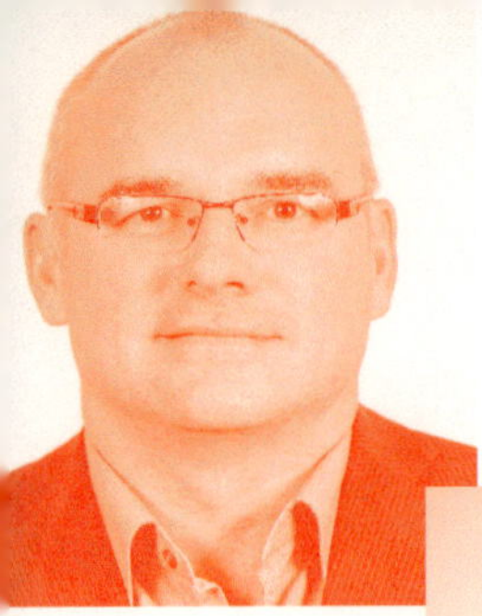
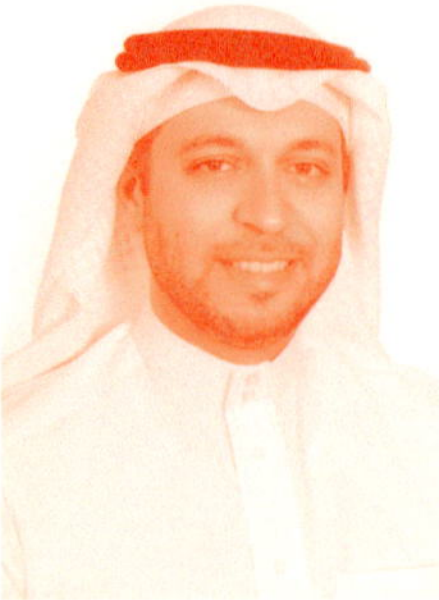
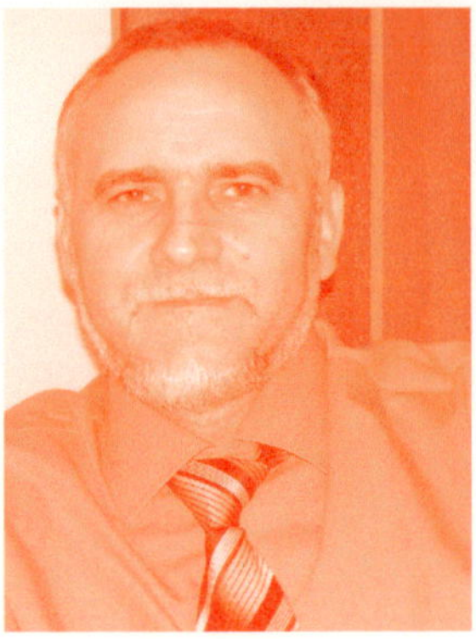
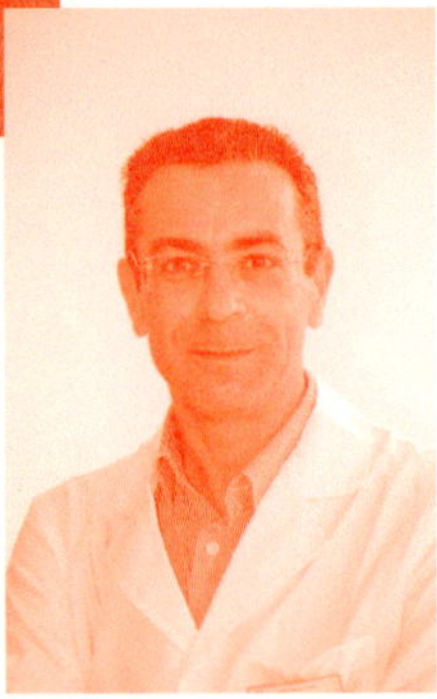
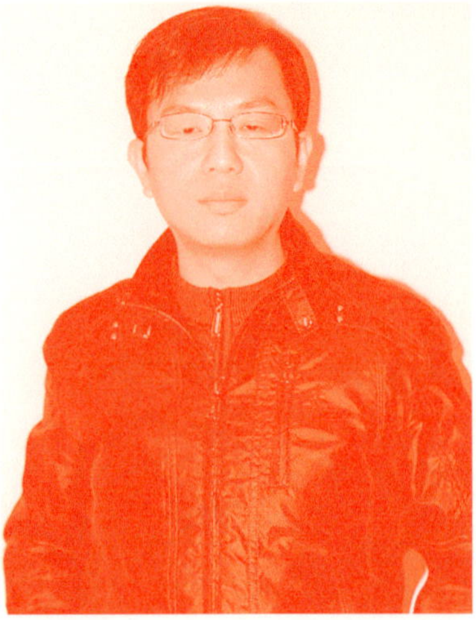
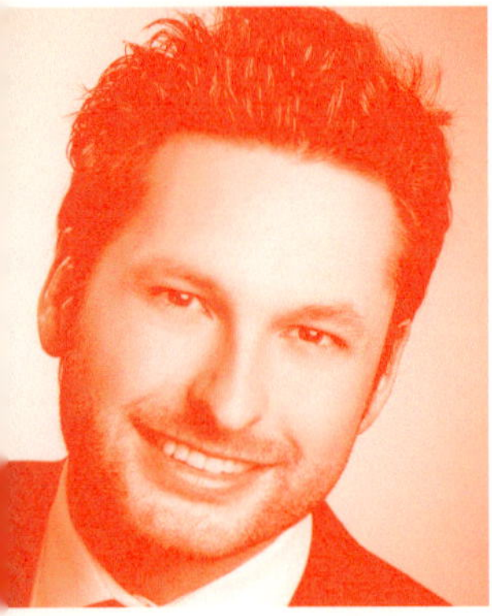
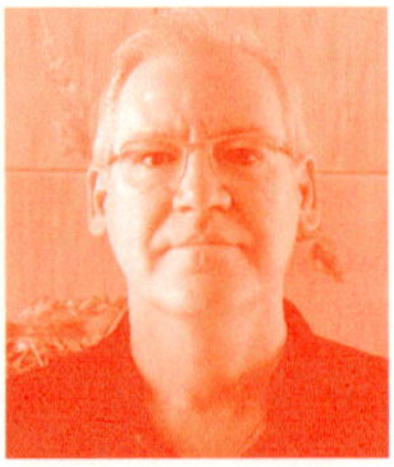

IntechOpen

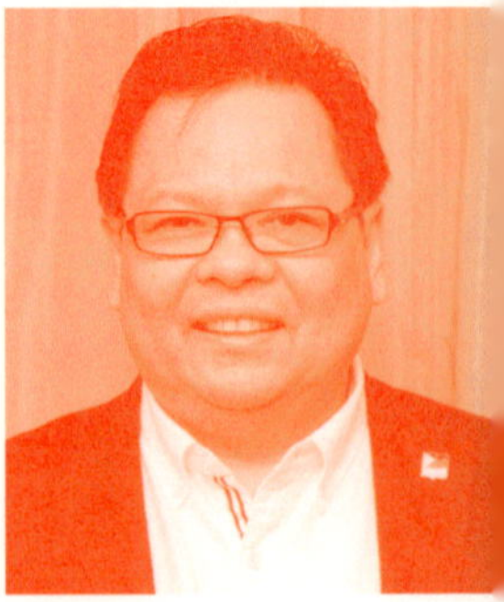
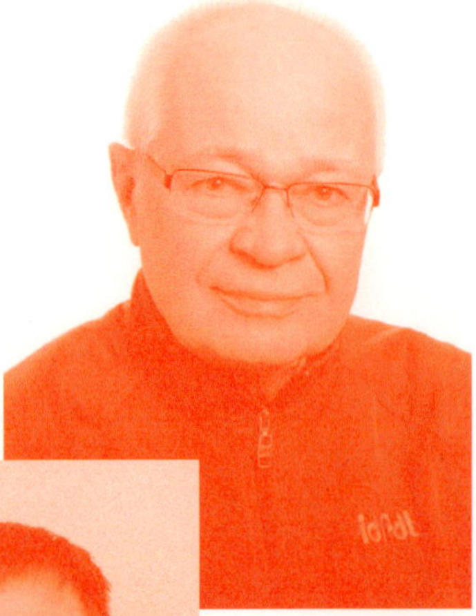
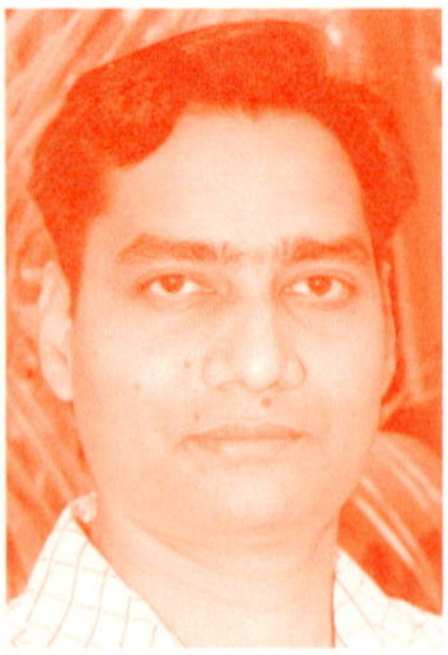
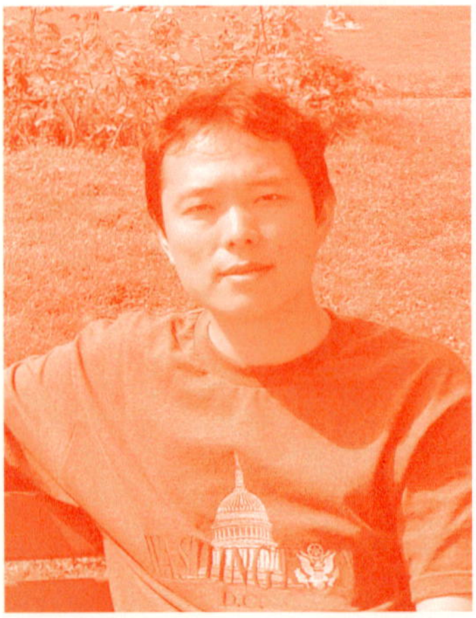
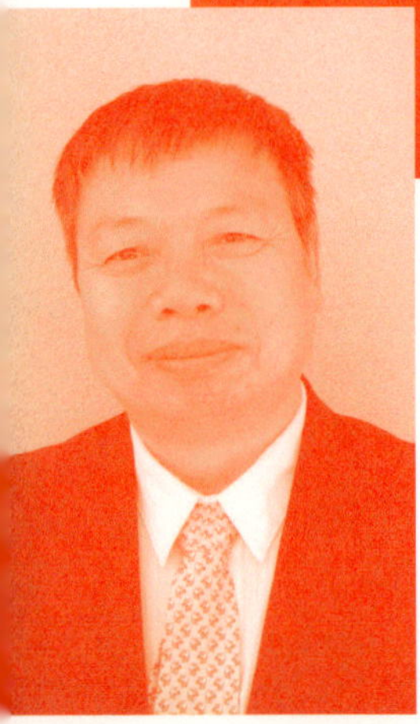
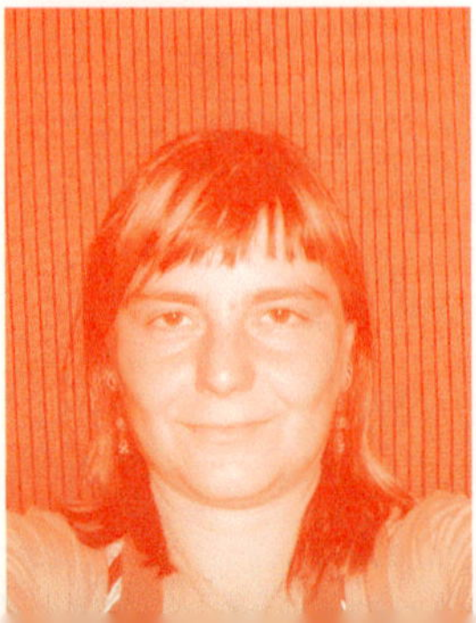

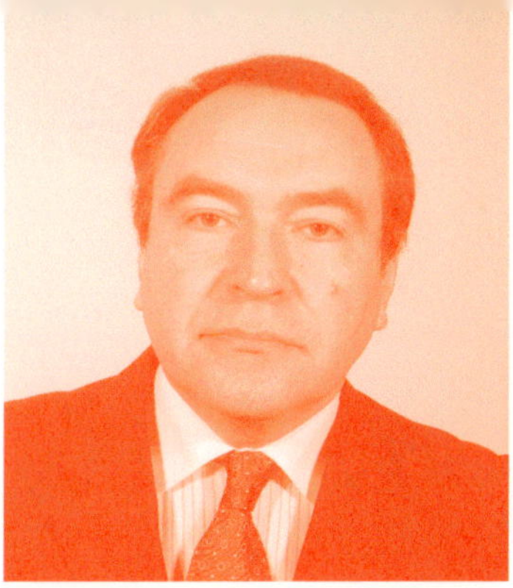
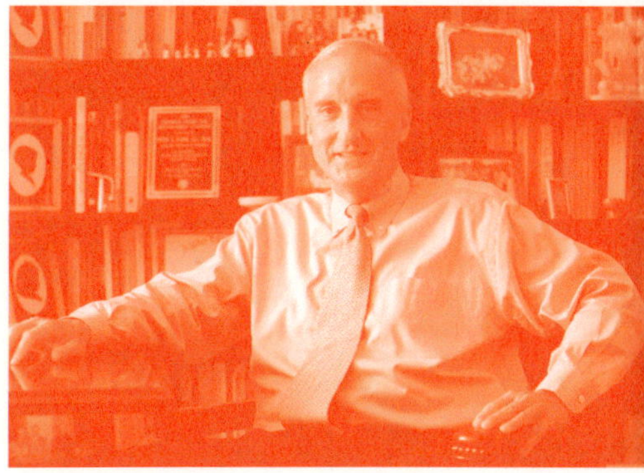
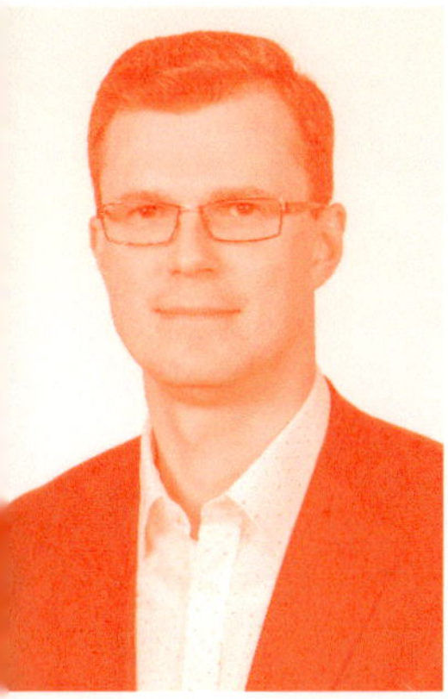
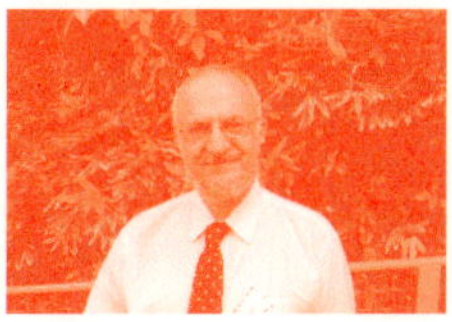
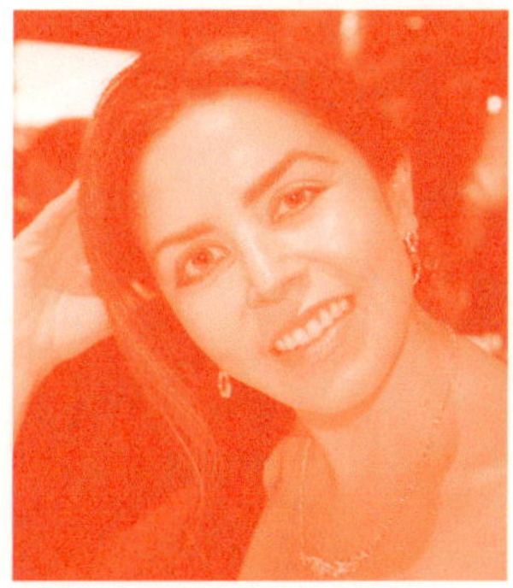

Supporting open minds since 2005

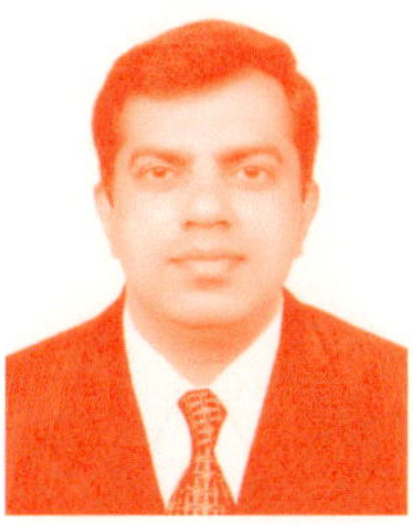
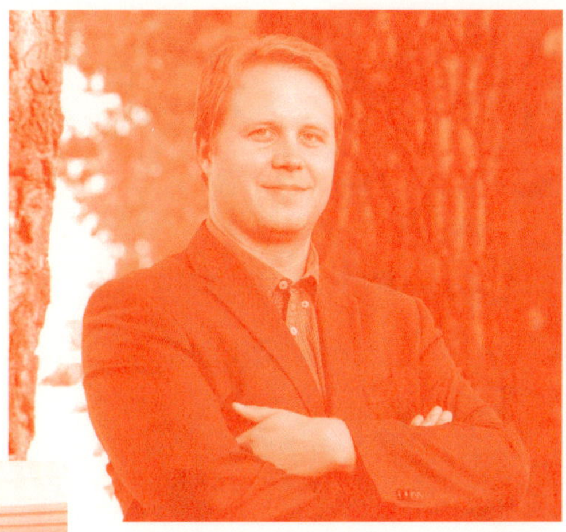
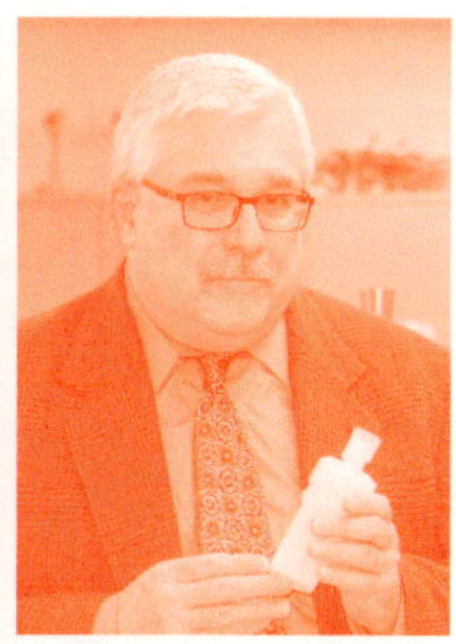
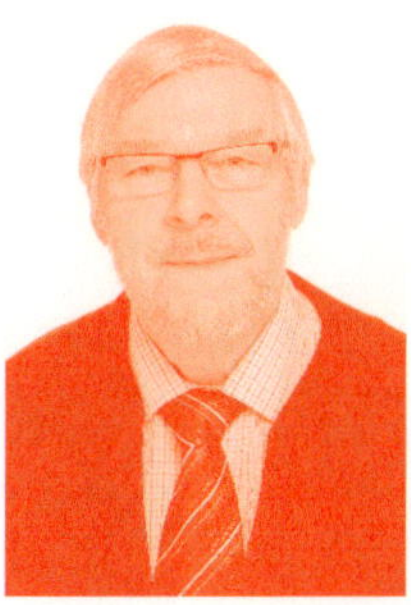
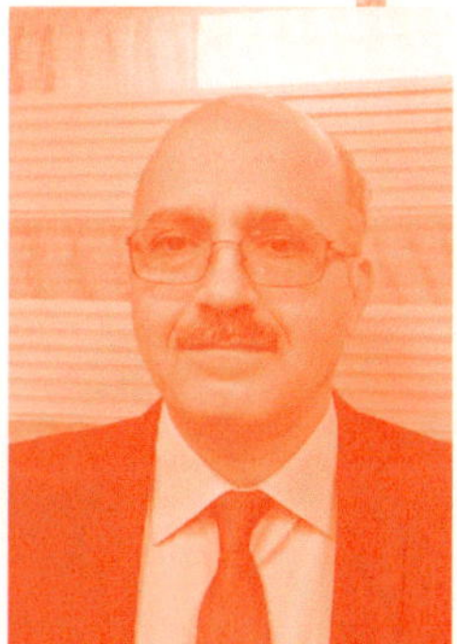
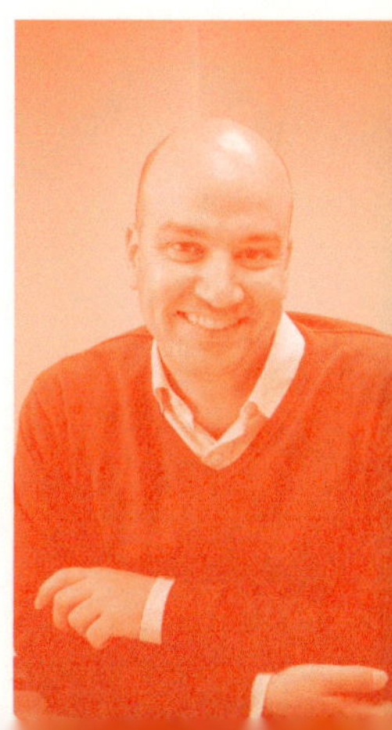
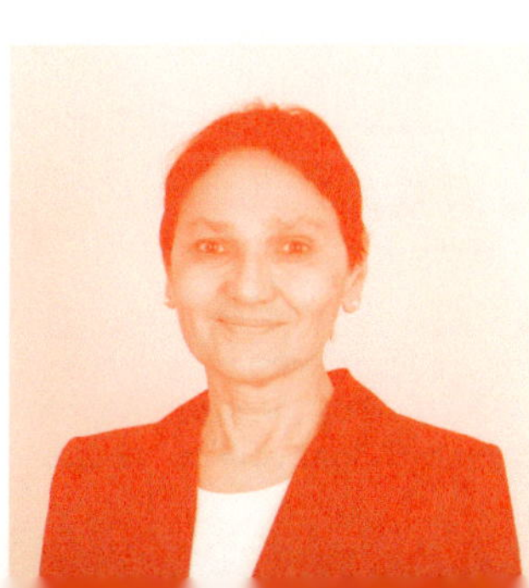

Psychology of Health - Biopsychosocial Approach
http://dx.doi.org/10.5772/intechopen.79036
Edited by Simon George Taukeni

Contributors
Ludmila Fialova, Kenechukwu C. C Onyekwelu, Dinara Adjablaeva, Irene Calesini, Vanessa Ferreira, Rosana Magalhães, Robert Motta, Carla Giambrone, Simon George Taukeni

First published in London, United Kingdom, 2019 by IntechOpen
IntechOpen is the global imprint of INTECHOPEN LIMITED, registered in England and Wales, registration number: 11086078, 7th floor, 10 Lower Thames Street, London, EC3R 6AF, United Kingdom
Printed in Croatia

British Library Cataloguing-in-Publication Data
A catalogue record for this book is available from the British Library

Additional hard and PDF copies can be obtained from orders@intechopen.com

Psychology of Health - Biopsychosocial Approach
Edited by Simon George Taukeni
p. cm.
Print ISBN 978-1-83880-217-2
Online ISBN 978-1-83880-218-9
eBook (PDF) ISBN 978-1-83962-636-4

For EU product safety concerns:
IN TECH d.o.o., Prolaz Marije Krucifikse Kozulić 3, 51000 Rijeka, Croatia, info@intechopen.com or visit our website at intechopen.com.

Meet the editor

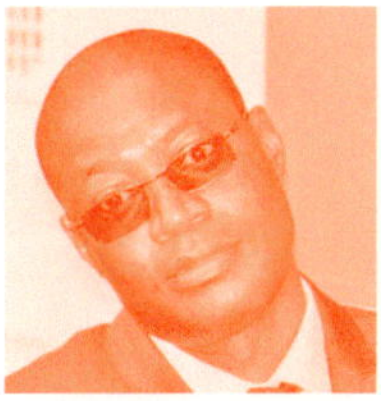

Dr. Simon George Taukeni is a Namibian academic, researcher, author, and editor. Dr. Taukeni is a former post-doctoral fellow at the University of Fort Hare. He holds a Doctor of Philosophy (Ph.D.) in education and two Master Degrees, namely: Master of Public Health and Master of Education from the University of Fort Hare in South Africa. He holds a Specialized Postgraduate Diploma in Special Education and a Bachelor of Education degree from the University of Namibia. To date, Simon has published four books and fourteen articles in accredited journals. He has attended a number of conferences and seminars locally and internationally. His areas of interest are in psychology, public health, and research.

Contents

Preface **III**

Chapter 1 **1**
Introductory Chapter: Bio-Psychosocial Model of Health
by Simon George Taukeni

Chapter 2 **9**
Physiology of Human Birth and Mental Disease
by Irene Calesini

Chapter 3 **25**
Assessing Quality of Life in Children and Adolescents Diagnosed with Pulmonary Tuberculosis
by Dinara Adjablaeva

Chapter 4 **35**
Ethanol
by Kenechukwu C. Onyekwelu

Chapter 5 **51**
Health Education and Lifestyles in the Czech Republic
by Ludmila Fialova

Chapter 6 **69**
The Role of Exercise in Reducing PTSD and Negative Emotional States
by Robert Motta

Chapter 7 **81**
Social Inequalities, Poverty and Obesity
by Vanessa Alves Ferreira and Rosana Magalhães

Chapter 8 **91**
Let Them See You Sweat: Integrating Yoga and Well-Being
by Carla A. Giambrone

Preface

This book aims to add knowledge to the field of health sciences and public health in particular. The focus is mainly on health psychology; namely the bio-psychosocial approach as a way to embrace health promotion, illness prevention, and health maintenance. The bio-psychosocial approach has contributed immensely to the field of health psychology. As a discipline, health psychology aims to examine how biological, psychological, and social factors influence people's behavior regarding their health status. The psychology of health is a specialty within the discipline of psychology concerned with individual behaviors and lifestyles affecting physical health. In the book by Sarafino (2008:11), the following goals of health psychology were presented:

- Promote and maintain health
- Prevent and treat illness
- Identify the causes and diagnosis correlates of health, illness and related dysfunction
- Analyse and improve health care systems and health policy.

The recognition of health psychology as a designated field is widely acknowledged. The relationship between mind and body and the effect of one upon the other has been widely debated amongst philosophers, psychologists, and physiologists. Central to the debate has been the question: **Why many people do not do what they know is in their best interest and why some people are more open to the adoption of healthy habits than others?** This is the key question that drives health psychologists to explore and influence lifestyles and behaviors that are conducive or detrimental to good health at the population level. This book is therefore in support of a consistent focus on the role of knowledge in informing people of the risks to themselves that certain behaviors can engender. I acknowledge the good work done by all the authors who contributed to this book. I hope that the readers, especially students, academics, researchers, and other professionals in Health Sciences and related fields, will learn the best practices as provided in the book. The specific chapters included in this book are as follows:

- Introductory Chapter: Bio-Psychosocial Model of Health
- Physiology of Human Birth and Mental Disease
- Assessing Quality of Life in Children and Adolescents Diagnosed with Pulmonary Tuberculosis
- Ethanol
- Health Education and Lifestyle in Czech Republic

- The Role of Exercise in Reducing PTSD and Negative Emotional States
- Social Inequalities, Poverty and Obesity
- Let Them See You Sweat: Integrating Yoga and Well-Being

Simon George Taukeni
University of Namibia,
Namibia

Chapter 1

Introductory Chapter: Bio-Psychosocial Model of Health

Simon George Taukeni

1. Introduction

Health psychology explores different ways in the pursuit of getting people to embrace health promotion, illness prevention and health maintenance. As a speciality, health psychology examines how biological, psychological and social factors influence people's behaviour about their health status. The aim of this chapter is to examine possible contributory connections between bio-psychosocial factors and health at the population level. The book explores bio-psychosocial model which can help individuals to develop and maintain healthy lifestyles so as to promote good health and prevent illness. Friedman and Adler [1] noted that the original bio-psychosocial model shaped not only research and theory on health but also the development of health psychology.

2. Definitions

2.1 Health

Kazarian and Evans [2] suggest that people commonly think about health in terms of an absence of (1) objective signs that the body is not functioning properly and (2) subjective symptoms of disease or injury, such as pain or nausea. World Health Organization defined health as 'a state of complete physical, mental and social well-being and not merely the absence of disease or infirmity' (WHO, 1946 cited in [3]:4). Some health psychologists defined health as a positive state of physical, mental and social well-being not simply the absence of injury or disease that varies over time along a continuum [4]. At the wellness end of the continuum, health is the dominant state. At the other end of the continuum, the dominant state is illness or injury, in which destructive processes produce characteristic signs, symptoms or disabilities [4]. For further detail, see **Figure 1**.

2.2 Health psychology

Health psychology is a speciality within the discipline of psychology concerned with individual behaviours and lifestyles affecting physical health. The discipline strives to enhance health, prevent and treat disease, identify risk factors and improve the healthcare system public opinion regarding health issues [5]. Matarazzo in 1980 (as cited in [3]:4) offered a definition of health psychology which has become widely accepted:

> *Health psychology is the aggregate of the specific educational, scientific and professional contributions of the discipline of psychology to the promotion and maintenance of health, the prevention and treatment of illness, the identification of*

etiologic and diagnostic correlates of health, illness and related dysfunction, and the analysis and improvement of the health care system and health policy formation.

2.3 The goals of health psychology

Sarafino ([4]:11) mentioned the following goals of health psychology as to:

- Promote and maintain health
- Prevent and treat illness
- Identify the causes and diagnosis correlates of health, illness and related dysfunction
- Analyse and improve healthcare systems and health policy

2.4 Background of health psychology to public health

The recognition of health psychology as a designated field is widely acknowledged. The relationship between mind and body and the effect of one upon the other has always been a controversial topic amongst philosophers, psychologists and physiologists. Within psychology, the development of the study of psychosomatic disorders owes much to Freud [3]. It has been observed in the recent studies that more deaths are caused now by heart disease, cancer and strokes which are by-product of changes in lifestyles in the twentieth century. Psychologists can be instrumental in investigating and influencing lifestyles and behaviours which are conducive or detrimental to good health [3].

2.5 Health behaviours

Health behaviour is part of maintaining a healthy lifestyle and avoiding ill health. These are known as protective health behaviours. Health protective behaviours include the following categories:

- Environmental hazard avoidance—avoiding areas of pollution or crime.
- Harmful substance avoidance—not smoking or drinking alcohol.
- Health practices—sleeping enough, eating sensibly and so forth.
- Preventive health care—dental check-ups and smear tests.
- Safety practices—repairing things, keeping first aid kits and emergency telephone numbers handy.

Although most of us are familiar with the need to engage in these health behaviours, only a few of us actually do so, and that is what we need to work on to remind people of adopting a better health lifestyles. Many other researchers such as Berg (1976 as cited in Pitts, 1998) asserted that most people are aware of which health behaviours should be engaged in; however, they frequently do not do so, and they instead do engage in activities which they know to be harmful to their health. It is this cantankerousness which psychologists have spent a great deal of time examining. The dilemma for health psychologists is to explain why some or many people do

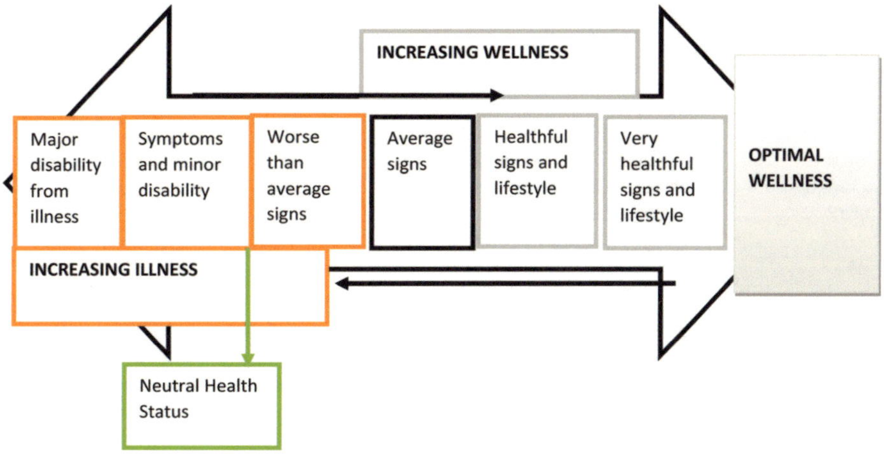

Figure 1.
Health (source: adopted from Sarafino [4]).

not do what they know is in their own best interest to do and why some people are more amenable to the adoption of healthy habits than others.

This chapter is therefore in support of a consistent focus on the role of knowledge in informing people of the risks to themselves that certain behaviours can engender. Pitts [3] reported studies that examining a range of issues relevant to health such as smoking, drug-taking, medical checks and adopting safer sex have fairly consistently shown that knowledge, by itself, does not lead to behaviour change. The only question left to ask is: So what is required, other than knowledge, to persuade people to look after their health? This question is the guiding principle to understand the role of health psychology in persuading people to look after their health informed by bio-psychosocial model.

2.6 Models of health

It is generally recognized that there are two models of health, namely, biomedical and bio-psychosocial models. Biomedical model focuses on treatment and elimination of symptoms, while bio-psychosocial model focuses on individual's perception of their symptoms and how they and their families respond to symptoms they are experiencing [6]. Also Deacon [7] asserts that under the biomedical model, illnesses were understood as having physiological aetiologies that were diagnosed through distinct biochemical markers and were to be treated through physical interventions. This chapter however is primarily focusing only on the bio-psychosocial models of health. Its founder, Engel [8], discovered that bio-psychosocial model represents the contribution of biological, psychological and social factors in determining health. **Table 1** shows the differences between the two models.

Within health psychology one model that has enjoyed considerable popularity is the 'stress-diathesis' model (Steptoe cited in [3]) which is currently called bio-psychosocial model. This model was first described by G.L. Engel in 1977. It emphasizes the interactive effect of environment and individual vulnerability (genetic and psychological characteristics) factors upon health [3]. According to bio-psychosocial model, psychological, physical and social threats present demands upon an individual's resources and capacity for coping which give rise to physiological reactions involving the autonomic nervous system (ANS) and endocrine and immune system of the body.

The effects include both short-term and long-term components, and these may have consequences on health depending upon the individual's predisposition or

Focal area	Biomedical model	Bio-psychosocial model
What causes illness?	Biological factors (chemical imbalances, bacteria, viruses and genetic predisposition)	Biological (virus), psychological (beliefs, behaviour) and social (unemployment)
Who is responsible for illness?	Individuals are regarded as victims of some external force causing internal changes. Because illness is seen as a result of biological changes beyond their control, individuals are not seen as responsible for their illness	Individuals should be held responsible for his/her health and illness
How should illness be treated?	Through vaccination, surgery, chemotherapy and radiotherapy, all of which aim to change the physical state of the body	The whole person should be treated, e.g. behaviour change, change in beliefs and coping strategies and compliance with medical recommendations
Who is responsible for treatment?	The responsibility for treatment rests with the medical profession	The focus is the whole person to be treated not just their physical illness; the patient is therefore responsible for their treatment (e.g. taking the medication or changing their behaviour)
What is the relationship between health and illness?	Health and illness are seen as qualitatively different—you are either healthy or ill—there is no continuum between the two	Health and illness exist on a continuum. Individuals progress along this continuum from health to illness and back again
What is the relationship between the mind and the body?	The mind and body function independently of each other. In other words, the mind and body are separate entities	The focus is on an interaction between the mind and the body. The mind and body interact
What is the role of psychology in health and illness?	Illness may have psychological consequences, but not psychological causes (e.g. cancer may cause unhappiness, but mood is not seen as related to either the onset or progression of the cancer)	Psychological factors not only as possible consequences of illness but as contributing to it at all stages along the continuum from healthy to being ill

Table 1.
Comparing biomedical and bio-psychosocial models of health.

vulnerability to adverse effects. Vulnerable individuals develop chronic allostatic reactions such as reduced immunocompetence or exaggerated sympathetic activation of the ANS or increased secretion of adrenal hormones. Physiological reactions of these types have been implicated in the development of many disease states, including cancers, cardiovascular diseases and other non-communicable diseases susceptibility to infections [3]. The following section presents the strengths and critical views of bio-psychosocial model.

2.7 Strengths of bio-psychosocial model

Bio-psychosocial model benefits the patients and healthcare system as revealed by research [8–14]:

- Guiding application of medical knowledge to the needs of each patient.
- Improved patient satisfaction, better adherence to prescriptions, more maintained behaviour change, better physical and psychological health and less of a tendency to initiate malpractice litigations.

- Development and application of techniques to reduce health risk behaviour.
- Reduce multiple visits and admission into hospitals.
- Individuals with health challenges are acknowledged to be active participants in the recovery process and good health, rather than mere passive victims.
- Increase efficiency of care by reducing unnecessary prescription of drugs (i.e. diabetes and other chronic conditions).
- Development of psychological techniques in the strengthening of immune reaction to illness.
- Bio-psychosocial model can be used as a predictor of pain and other psychosocial problems resulting into development appropriate prevention and intervention strategies.
- Improvement of communication between health staff and the patients.
- Development and introduction of programmes of life quality improvement for chronic patients, physically disabled individuals and the elderly patients.
- A significant influence on contemporary understanding of mental health difficulties.
- Development and application of psychosocial support for the terminally ill patients and their families.

2.8 Critical views of bio-psychosocial model

A list of critical views of bio-psychosocial model has been noted in literature [9, 10, 12, 15–18] as follows:

- Time-consuming and expensive apply.
- It requires more information be gathered during the assessment about an individual's socioeconomic status, culture, religion, as well as psychological factors that might affect the individual's condition.
- There is a lack of theoretical basis of bio-psychosocial model and scientific evidence to support the model.
- The complex relations between causes and effects of biological, psychological and social factors to influence the state of health and or occurrence of diseases.
- The holistic nature of the bio-psychosocial model makes it a luxury many healthcare systems in resource-poor settings cannot afford.
- Insufficient training opportunities or financial resources available to support the existence of multidisciplinary teams consisting of psychiatrists, clinical psychologists, mental health nurses and social welfare workers to allow for a full understanding of the biological, psychological and social factors involved in individual's condition.

- The model's failure to provide straightforward guidelines for clinical treatment or rules for prioritization in clinical practice.

- Medical students receive very limited amount of content in psychosocial subjects compared to biomedical-oriented courses.

3. Conclusion

The focus of this chapter was mainly on integrating bio-psychosocial model in public health discipline. Authors like Nadir et al. [12] found that bio-psychosocial model has been a mainstay in the ideal practice of modern medicine. It is attributed to improve patient care, compliance and satisfaction and to reduce physician-patient conflict. Both strengths and critical views of bio-psychosocial model were presented in the chapter. Even though it appears that patients and healthcare system are likely to benefit from the utilization of bio-psychosocial model, further research is still needed to determine whether or not bio-psychosocial model is a workable model in healthcare system to benefit all patients. In particular, more knowledge about how psychosocial factors can influence health and disease remain unclear to most public health professionals.

Author details

Simon George Taukeni
University of Namibia, Namibia

*Address all correspondence to: staukeni@gmail.com

References

[1] Friedman HS, Adler NE. The history and background of health psychology. In: Friedman HS, Silver RC, editors. Foundations of Health Psychology. NY: Oxford University Press; 2007. pp. 3-18

[2] Kazarian SS, Evans DR. Health psychology and culture: Embracing the 21st century. In: Kazarian SS, Evans ER, editors. Handbook of Cultural Health Psychology. San Diego: Academic Press; 2001. pp. 3-43

[3] Pitts M. An introduction to health psychology. In: Pitts M, Phillips K, editors. The Psychology of Health. Routledge: Wadsworth Publishing; 1998

[4] Sarafino EP. Health Psychology: Biopsychosocial Interactions. 6th ed. New Jersey: John Wiley & Sons; 2008

[5] Brannon L, Feist J. Health Psychology: An Introduction to Behaviour and Health. 5th ed. Belmont, CA: Wadsworth Thomson; 2004

[6] Morof I, Lubkin PD, Larsen P. Chronic Illness: Impact and Interventions. Boston: Jones and Bartlett; 2002

[7] Deacon BJ. The biomedical model of mental disorder. A critical analysis of its validity, utility and effects on psychotherapy research. Clinical Psychology Review. 2013;**33**:846-861

[8] Engel GL. The need for a new medical model: A challenge for biomedicine. Science. 1977;**196**:129-136

[9] Babalola E, Noel P, White R. The bio-psychosocial approach and global mental health: Synergies and opportunities. Indian Journal of Social Psychiatry. 2017;**33**:291-296

[10] Borrell-Carrió F, Suchman AL, Epstein RM. The bio-psychosocial model 25 years later: Principles, practice, and scientific inquiry. The Annals of Family Medicine. 2004;**2**:576-582

[11] Kamper SJ, Apeldoorn AT, Chiarotto A, Smeets RJ, Ostelo RW, Guzman J, et al. Multidisciplinary bio-psychosocial rehabilitation for chronic low back pain: Cochrane systematic review and meta-analysis. British Medical Journal. 2015;**350**:h444

[12] Nadir M, Hamza M, Mehmood N. Assessing the extent of utilization of bio-psychosocial model in doctor-patient interaction in public sector hospitals of a developing country. Indian Journal of Psychiatry. 2018;**60**(1):103-108

[13] Stewart M, Brown JB, Donner A, McWhinney IR, Oates J, Weston WW, et al. The impact of patient-centered care on outcomes. The Journal of Family Practice. 2000;**49**:796-804

[14] Williams GC, Frankel RM, Campbell TL, Deci EL. Research on relationship-centered care and healthcare outcomes from the Rochester bio-psychosocial program: A self-determination theory integration. Journal of Family System Health. 2000;**18**:79-90

[15] Armstrong D. Silence and truth in death and dying. Social Science & Medicine. 1987;**24**(8):651-657

[16] Gatchel RJ, Oordt MS. Clinical Health Psychology and Primary Care: Practical Advice and Clinical Guidance for Successful Collaboration. Washington, DC: American Psychological Association; 2012

[17] Lane RD. Is it possible to bridge the bio-psychosocial and biomedical models? Biopsychosocial Medicine. 2014;**8**:3

[18] Suls J, Rothman A. Evolution of the bio-psychosocial model: Prospects and challenges for health psychology. Health Psychology. 2004;**23**:119-125

Chapter 2

Physiology of Human Birth and Mental Disease

Irene Calesini

Abstract

This chapter elucidates the *physiology of birth* and the pathology of human mind in accordance with Massimo Fagioli's theory of human birth (1972). Human life and psychic activity begin at birth, with the reaction of the biological matter to light, an inanimate reality which is absent in the fetal condition. Thus a *capability to imagine* arises and will develop throughout life. The 'first human thinking' begins as an image and non-conscious mental activity. This dynamic is common to all human beings, without sexual or ethnic differences. Mental illness is a *disease* affecting the irrational, non-conscious dimension, determined by a deficiency of affection in early human relationships. Mental illness is not a condition men are destined to, but rather a pathology that can be treated and cured through psychodynamic psychotherapy, within a valid therapeutic human relationship. This theory and its psychotherapeutic approach could provide new perspectives and possibilities for healthcare services and prevention policies, to assure mental well-being.

Keywords: human birth theory, annulment pulsion, vitality, capability to react, capability to imagine, disappearance fantasy, mental health, mental illness, well-being, psychotherapy

1. Introduction

The aim of this chapter is to discuss the physiology and the pathology of the mind according to Massimo Fagioli's Human Birth Theory [1]. The aim of this theory is to explain the origin of human thought and the formation of mind physiology and pathology. Fagioli was an Italian neuropsychiatrist and psychotherapist most well known for his theory and psychotherapeutic practice, the Analisi Collettiva. This was a large psychotherapy group which began in 1975 and was carried uninterruptedly by Massimo Fagioli until December 2016. The 'Collective Analysis' represented a unique phenomenon in the worldwide psychotherapeutic practice, characterized by free sessions attended by a spontaneous inflow of people —more than 200 participants at each sitting—in which Fagioli continuously interpreted dreams within the specific framework of cure, training and research [2, 3]. In contrast to widespread psychoanalytic/psychiatric concepts and to classical anthropological/philosophical cultures that assert an original fragmentation and chaos of human mind, this theory affirms the native psychological health and the psyche-soma fusion at birth. More precisely, he describes and demonstrates the birth's physiology of mind and thought, starting from the human biological reality. The revolutionary importance of his theory lies in the discovery and formulation that human life and psychic activity begin at birth, with the reaction of the biological matter to light, an inanimate reality which is absent in the fetal condition. This concept is continually stressed throughout the whole author's work until his latest writings [4–6]. Consequently, according to this theory, the process leading to the primary formation of human thinking is independent of any influence exerted by other human beings, from neither the mother nor any transcendental entity. Birth has, on the contrary, only a specie-specific biological origin. Therefore, it is fundamental to clarify the dynamics that underlie the physiology of the mind in order to fully comprehend the onset of mental illness, which is not innate but acquired. In all human beings, body and mind are merged together at birth. In particular, the mind has both conscious and unconscious dimensions respectively controlled by conscious and non-conscious mechanisms. This concept is neither particularly widespread nor accepted in the field of psychiatry which still nowadays maintains a predominantly organicist approach, mainly focusing on consciousness, external behavior and cognitive abilities. However, it is important to consider non-conscious reality in order to accurately understand the functioning of human action and thought. As proposed and demonstrated by Massimo Fagioli in his large theoretical proposition and clinical praxis, it is pivotal to adopt a biological rather than a religious perspective when discussing mind physiology. Human birth physiology is equal for all human beings regardless gender, ethnicity and nationalities. Non-conscious dimension is the first reality to develop in human beings, arising at birth in the same dynamic that marks the beginning of human life. Soon after birth, the newborn will naturally look for another human being in order to find confirmations and to develop a personal and unaware knowledge arisen at birth: the existence of a valid relationship able to fulfill its needs not only for nourishment but also for love and affection [1]. This natural tendency to look and move toward a valid human relationship continues throughout all life playing a fundamental role, particularly during childhood up until adolescence. However, if a deficiency of affection is particularly present in the relationship with the mother or another significant adult during the first year of life, the hopeful certainty of a valid human relationship can be seriously compromised. According to this theory, a lack of affection during the first year of life must be considered as a postnatal pathogenic factor that can determine a similar lack of affection in the adolescent and later the onset of mental illness. In this case, if the adolescent suffers the consequences of a pathological relation, a connected pathogenic defensive mechanism (annulment pulsion, negation, and bramosy) will be addressed toward non valid human beings, causing dysfunctional or altered behaviors [1, 7, 8]. Moreover, we should consider that during this period the relationship with the opposite gender will play a relevant role in the adolescent's mental development. The Theory of Birth claims that mental illness is caused by specific and early pathogenic interhuman dynamics. They are an acquired condition and cannot be considered as an inherent constitutive feature. Nevertheless, they can be treated through psychotherapy within a valid therapeutic human relationship. In the following chapter, I will describe the physiological mechanism at the core of the body-mind formation at birth and also the most important pathological mechanisms that arise first in the non-conscious mind and only later manifest their effects with altered conscious thought, behavior and language.

2. Methods and analysis

The writing of this chapter is fundamentally and largely based on the wide scientific production of Professor Massimo Fagioli. In particular its content draws from the Theory of Birth with a specific attention to the formation of human thought, mind physiology and the onset and development of mental illness in early relationships. For what concerns the clinical methods and the therapeutic use of this theory in the psychotherapeutic intervention, I have made used not only of the author's theoretical writings but also of my direct experience of cure and formation which lasted 37 years in the Analisi Collettiva psychotherapy group. This large psychotherapy began as a spontaneous movement at the University of Rome in January 1975 and was carried uninterruptedly by Massimo Fagioli until December 2016. The 'Collective Analysis' was held at the University of Rome for the first 5 years and was then moved into a spacious private studio. This represents a unique phenomenon in the worldwide psychotherapeutic practice, characterized by free sessions attended by a spontaneous inflow of people—more than 200 participants at each sitting. At the beginning the session lasted 2 hours and the duration was then increased up to 4. At the core of any psychotherapy and in particular of this, lies the idea that every human being has been and is continuously affected by human relationships. Therefore mental reality can be changed and transformed in a human and therapeutic relationship. In this setting, the interpretation of oniric images was connected with the unconscious relationship with the therapist (transfert), the group and the broader social and cultural reality. This was a crucial aspect of the Theory. Oniric images are a non conscious form of thinking which can be understood, interpreted and verbalized, thanks to the therapist's personal sensibility and non-conscious reality. These qualities allow the therapist to understand what the patient is communicating through his/her dream by also perceiving the patient's non-verbal language and attitude. In this sense, the interpretation of dreams is founded on the psychotherapist's demand that violent unconscious dimensions (expressed by the patient through rage, envy and lack of affection) must be refused by the patient itself by making them disappear. The interpretation of one individual's dreams in front of other people allows many to recognize oneself in the dynamics interpreted. Therefore each individual by comprehending the interpretation of another patient can turn this into personal knowledge. The individual perceives that mental illness is not only a personal, neither incomprehensible nor incurable situation. This method has been applied in much smaller groups and in individual psychotherapies by many psychiatrists and psychotherapists that in addition to an academic formation in psychiatry and psychology have followed this story firstly as patients, together with other people.

3. Intrauterine condition

In the uterus, amniotic fluid in the homeostatic condition surrounds the fetus. This chemical and physical state guarantees the protection of the fetus from any external variation. In the darkness of this "before birth" condition there is no light stimulation. Although around the 22nd post conceptional week (PCW) visual connections are already partially formed, the sight function has not developed yet [9, 10]. Clinical experience and publications have shown that from the 23rd to 24th PCW, the fetus is capable of surviving without any developmental harm if adequately assisted with medical intensive treatment. This is what is defined as viability, a condition that implies not only being born alive but it is closely related to the concepts of capability of meaningful life and of reasonable period of survival [11]. Viability appears to be strictly related to the subplate zone which plays a major role in the structural development of connectivity and cerebral cortex neuromaturation [11]. The subplate is a transient compartment of the fetal telencephalic wall, placed under the cortical plate. This hosts the majority of fetal neurons and reaches a developmental peak around the 23rd–24th PWC. The subplate zone functions as a waiting compartment for growing cortical afferents, in particular thalamic-cortical connections, which play an important function in the somatic-sensory function.

These develop in the subplate zone, creating temporary synaptic circuits and normally wait months before being relocated in the cerebral cortex, their final target [10, 12, 13]. In the occipital zone, the subplate's main function is to organize the optical orientation columns. Moreover, this is an area of intense synaptic activity where endogenous stimuli trigger specific fetal electrical activities: the spontaneous transient activity (SATs), which can be traced through electroencephalography (EEG) [14]. Its role is to organize and structure neuronal nets in the fetal brain (the thalamus cortical connection) and to give origin to transient circuits. This activity ends at birth when the permanent cortical circuit and the externally driven cortical circuitry, situated in the cerebral cortex will be activated [12]. The subplate has a fundamental role in brain plasticity and some of its neurons survive after birth until adolescence and early adulthood as subcortical interstitial neurons of the gyral white matter [12]. In the subplate zone, excitatory neurons which work with the gamma-aminobutyric acid (GABA) are implied in the connectivity and cerebral cortex structure development. At birth, GABA will become the major neurotransmitter inhibitor (and will play this role for the whole life) determining a change in the cerebral electrical activity of the newborn. This switch is triggered by the retina light stimulation [15]. These scientific observations consistently support the Theory of Birth formulated by Massimo Fagioli. The concept of viability has been strictly related to capability to react to sensorial stimuli that will occur at birth [11]. Other author highlight how cortico-cortical and thalamo-cortical connections, the subplate, the SAT and the somatosensory reactivity are all present at the same time when the capability to survive has been reached at 23rd–24th PCW. This has been linked with what will occur after birth [16]. In particular the sensation experienced in contact with the amniotic fluid which is a fundamental prerequisite to realize what Fagioli called "memory fantasy" [1, 16]. When the fetus is in contact with the amniotic fluid, can the uterus be considered a closed system. At the same time the fetus's brain electrical activity has the only role to organize and structure neuronal networks. At birth this condition will completely change in the dramatic passage from the intrauterine condition to the external world: the organization and the fetal brain function will be modified. The subplate as guide and cytoarchitectonic structure disappears, the SATs frequencies decrease until their presence on the EEG disappears and regular waves, which are correlated with alive condition, will appear [12, 14]. The GABA neurotransmitter function changes as previously stated. Finally the external environment condition is now dramatically different for the newborn. This determines a drastic caesura between the intrauterine and the extra uterine condition.

4. Physiology at birth

In the intrauterine condition, the fetus is only a biological reality in contact with another biological substance; the amniotic fluid. There is no psychic activity in the uterus: mental activity will start at birth when irreversible changes occur both in the body and in the brain. In the homeostatic condition where no harmful stimuli are present, organs and apparatus developmental processes occur. Toward the end of pregnancy, from the 23rd to 24th PCW, the fetus has the possibility to survive when "coming to light", but until it is in the intrauterine condition it cannot be considered alive in terms of body and mind functioning. The fetus will become a human being when stimulated by light, an absolute new feature which will determine the activation of the brain. Whereas tactile stimulation is not new to the newborn as it was previously enveloped in the amniotic fluid of the intrauterine environment, light is a completely new stimulus. Recent studies have provided biological data that can be related to the psychic dynamic happening at birth and firstly theorized and described by Massimo Fagioli in 1972. Moreover, several authors have interpreted these biological data in the light of this theory [11, 16]. In the central nervous system the retina, through the pupil, is the only part of the cerebral matter open to external stimuli. At birth, photo-retinal stimulation triggers an immediate pulsional reaction specific to humans which is a specific biological feature of *Homo sapiens*, denominated by Fagioli as annulment pulsion (pulsione di annullamento) [1, 4–6, 17]. Recent scientific studies have shown that a single photon is sufficient for the activation of retinal cells [18]. As soon as it passes through the pupil and hits the retina, light immediately determines the brain's activation. This happens within a timeframe of the order of femtoseconds, so as to trigger the chain of chemical and physical events leading to the activation of brain circuits [19]. It has been studied that at birth the activation of the brain through visual connection and occipital cortex stimulation is faster than other cortical stimulation nervous pathway for the activation of vital processes such as respiration [20]. In addition, it has been shown how light is involved in the functional change of the GABA neurotransmitter at birth [15]. The newborn experiences a dramatic change, passing from the homeostatic condition in the amniotic fluid to the completely new extrauterine condition. The newborn reacts to the aggressiveness of the external non-human world (such as light, air, noise, cold) by closing the eyes and 'making it dark'. By doing so the newborn makes mentally disappear the external inanimate material world and at the same time, it would tend make itself disappear too. This is the pulsional defensive and non-conscious reaction defined by Fagioli as annulment pulsion. Through this pulsion, the mind of the newborn by wishing of returning to the previous stage makes both the external world and itself disappear. However, this cannot happen as the brain has been activated by light and the mind is now functioning together with the body. The fetus does not exist and neither the conditions that allowed its existence. The newborn cannot return into the darkness of the intrauterine condition. If the newborn managed to make itself "disappear" as a body-mind reality, it would not attach to the breast, and this wouldn't permit a natural movement toward another human being. The newborn would die. Thus, it is not possible for the newborn to annul its birth because something impedes this pulsion to turn into auto-destruction: vitality [1]. Vitality, a specie-specific human feature, has its roots in the capability to react that develops at 24th PCW and is strictly connected to the biological reality of the body. At birth the capability to react arises in the newborn, making possible the reaction to the light stimuli. This reaction is the annulment pulsion which simultaneously activates vitality. At birth vitality and the annulment pulsion are merged together. This latter does not exist independently, as it occurs in serious mental illness on a non-conscious level. Moreover, as it was previously stated, this would lead to the newborn's death. The fusion between vitality and annulment pulsion becomes 'fantasia di sparizione' or disappearance fantasy [1]. This formulation was theorized and firstly published by Massimo Fagioli in 1972. Since then, this theory has been confirmed by further investigation and research. The author brings together two concepts that identify two inherently and antithetical human features. Fantasy is related to imagination and therefore to the creation of something that did not exist before. However, 'disappearance' implies that something that existed before now does not exist anymore. This concept may sound contradictory but it is indeed able to express a creative act that happens without awareness in the newborn (which is a non-conscious act). Similarly, at birth, the newborn, by making the external non-human world disappear, creates the first image-idea of itself. This is the first creative act of the newborn, the first human thought. As the external inanimate world disappears in the newborn's mind, vitality allows the formation of a first undefined image. (Fagioli called this first image inconscio mare calmo, providing a clear visual image). At birth, the newborn realizes a first sensorial memory of the experience had in the previous homeostatic condition. According to Fagioli's theorization, in the first moments of life the newborn realizes a memory-fantasy of the experience had in the intrauterine condition, from the sensation with the skin in contact with the amniotic fluid, (memory-fantasy of the sensation had before), and a first image of itself as 'libidinal and psychic self'; at the same time, the newborn by recreating in its mind the condition of wellbeing and calmness previously experienced, imagines the existence of another human being similar to itself. In those first moments of the newborn's life from the pulsional and vital rejection of the inanimate world, the certainty of an existing breast arises; that is, a human being similar to itself to whom to direct its feeling. In conclusion, the newborn makes the external world disappear, but not itself or its natural tendency toward another human being. This is the psychodynamic result of the first reaction to the external non-human world. For further references we suggest Chapter 2 in [1]. It is important to reaffirm that the annulment pulsion at birth is not isolated as it is merged with vitality. Together they become disappearance fantasy, which is creative and not destructive. According to Fagioli specification, these two specific human features the annulment pulsion and vitality, arising immediately in 'coming to light', make the newborn indifferent to the inanimate external world and at the same time enable the creation of the capability to imagine [21, 22]. This capability to imagine is a fundamental human dimension throughout all life. Indeed a loss or alteration of this dimension is founded in most psychiatric pathologies as I will further explain in the following paragraphs. The capability to imagine is an exclusive human characteristic, which begins at birth and develops throughout life. The first human thinking, which begins as image and non-conscious mental activity, represents the basis of any creative activity. The capability to imagine is realized at birth in the short span of time between the light stimulation and the subsequent pulsional reaction with the activation of the respiratory muscles by the central nervous system. Physiologically it occurs in those first instants of life when the newborn appears to be inert and it still not crying nor breathing. Only after this short span of time the newborn wails and moves. This is a common experience in the delivery room: a suspended moment, a bunch of seconds when the newborn is still and not wailing. However, as previously explained the light has already hit the retina therefore the brain has been activated and the mind is functioning. Although the newborn appears still and silent, it is already alive and human. This is how the biological formation of human psyche occurs. To sum up, **light is the absolute new feature. Annulment pulsion toward non human reality and vitality determine disappearance fantasy as the capability to imagine, the creation of the first internal image and the certainty of an existing breast.** The 'Human Birth theory' proves that the first act in the newborn's life is an autonomous psychic act. This is an individual creation arising from the biological reality through the reaction to light. Human life starts, when at birth mental activity begins. In our whole life, this activity will never cease, neither during the night. It will stop only at the death of the individual. Therefore, the lifetime of a human being is all comprised within an interval that starts when light activates the brain, while the end corresponds to the cessation of mental activity. During the night human thoughts will express themselves through images as non-conscious thought. The interpretation of oniric images and the presence or lack of affection concealed in these images is at the core of psychotherapy according to the Theory of Birth.

5. The interhuman relationship

It is a commonly accepted notion that since the early months of life infants are able to make connections with their surrounding world. Therefore contrary to what

Freud affirmed [23], they cannot be considered as isolated, autoerotic and narcissistic beings [24]. Nowadays it is a proven fact that cognitive development is affected by early social relationship and by the newborn activity. Moreover, recent studies carried by Murray have confirmed the idea that infants begin to make connection to the world since the very beginning [25]. This study, based on observation and experimental approach, demonstrates the early communication ability shown by infants. As early as the first month of life, the newborn smiles without being able to distinguish to whom. At the same time the newborn is able to interact with other human beings approaching its visual area, through visual contact. During the second month, although the vision is not completely formed, the infant begins to make visual connection with the mother's face. (Visual acuity gradually develops over the first year of life and it will be completely formed at the age of two. In the earliest months of life the baby can differentiate only lights, shadows and sharp movements). According to Murray, during the second month of life the intersubjective primary phase begins. During this time the infant starts to smile and to socially interact with his/her parents that can now recognize their infant as human. Moreover at this stage, mirror neurons and the parent's tendency to imitate sounds and gestures of their infant play a fundamental role. These factors help to develop a sense of reciprocity and trust. Through their careful presence parents can provide love and affection to their infants, addressing their needs and guaranteeing a safe attachment [25]. It is well known that early experiences during the first year of life will have a major impact on the onset of mental illness during adolescence and early adulthood. B. Beebe has confirmed the existence of four type of attachment (secure, avoidant, ambivalent, disorganized) which had been previously identified by her mentor Stern. In her recent work is highlighted how a disorganized attachment during the first year of life can have dramatic consequence in adulthood, resulting in serious mental illness. Beebe also hypothesizes the importance of mirror neurons in early relational experiences [26]. Although these relevant experimental studies and observations should be considered the object of further research, we think that the core of this discussion does not lie in the behavioral and emotional mirroring. What is central is rather the infant's need to find confirmation of its feeling and identity in the interhuman relationship. Obviously it is necessary to consider that developmental processes, cognitive and emotional acquisition and the act of processing experiences are directly related to biological activities, neurofunctional mechanism and remodeling of the neural networking. The latter is still partly unknown and we do not intend to deny nor underestimate their role believing that they should be considered object of further investigation. We should remember that brain neural plasticity reaches a peak during the first year of life and continues developing until the age of 18–30 [10, 12]. However, we must point out the limits founded in the approaches previously mentioned. Although they highlight the importance of interhuman dynamics during the preverbal period and take into account the centrality of nonverbal communication (gesture, body posture, facial and vocal expression, physical or non-physical contact), they still mainly consider a relational context in which adult behavior and consciousness are the main agents. These act together with the primitive infant consciousness, which is considered as "internal operative models" shaped on the base of experience [26]. One of the major limits of these neuropsychological approaches lies in the complete absence of research on the origin of irrational and non conscious mind. According to the theory of birth, the infant non-conscious mind is the first to be formed in human beings and for a quite a long time will be the only function. The non-conscious mind is strictly connected to the infant body. In fact, body and mind are born together in "coming to light" with a drastic separation that marks the end of the conditions that guaranteed the fetus existence. We should recall how investigating the human birth

dynamic can be fundamental in order to understand how mind's individuality and sociality are formed. Since birth, the infant is able to establish a relationship with other human beings with its all human reality. A few moments after birth, the cold inanimate reality does not exist and the search for human relationships begins. This is a crucial moment for every human being. As previously explained, because of the human birth dynamic, the newborn processes and develops a 'certainty of an existing breast'. This is not a rational certainty but rather an irrational, unconscious natural tendency toward another human being. While in the earliest moment of life, mental reality is shaped in the relation (refusal) with the inanimate world; firstly, light. Soon after, once the First Self is formed, in order to live, the search for the other starts. By 'living', we consider at the same time a material and psychic life. In fact, since this moment the infant development is strictly connected to both cognitive and affective growth. If the newborn is not physically nourished it dies. However a child that receives physical nourishment but is left alone, not warmly welcomed or taken care will manifest signs of severe depression until death [27].
I would like to further specify that according to the Massimo Fagioli Theory the newborn once born is neither undifferentiated nor shapeless. This means that it won't acquire an emotional and cognitive shape through the relationship with the mother. On the contrary, it is in the sharp caesura happening at birth that the newborn separate oneself from the mother and the intrauterine condition. In doing so an irrational mind is first created in the interaction with the inanimate world. Only in a second moment the newborn will establish a rapport with the mother (or with another significant human being). The newborn will naturally establish a relation of trust that characterizes the primitive and originary human sociality. This arises from the process occurring at birth in which the newborn without being aware is sure of the existence of a breast. The adult's duty is to be physically and psychologically ready to give warmth and nourishment, in order to confirm this infant intuition. The warm voice of the mother or another significant being, the harmony of the words heard, the lullabies sang, the care received and the affection given will physically transmit invisible forms of affection. The newborn feels and perceives the internal non-conscious reality of the caregiver. The caregiver's unconscious reality will be based on love and interest for the newborn if this is considered as a human being in all respects. On the contrary, the caregiver will be merely addressing the newborn's physical needs if this is uniquely seen as a body to nourish and to be look after. The caregiver's inner reality and their psychic wellbeing are fundamental for the healthy development of the newborn. It is also important for clinicians to consider what occurs in the adults' non-conscious mind during the interaction with the newborn immediately after birth and during the earliest years of life. During the infant development, cognitive acquisitions go hand in hand with emotional experiences. Consciousness comes only later when physical senses mature and the cerebral connection are completely formed, thanks to evident brain plasticity now widely demonstrated. Therefore mirroring and imitational processes are not key in the relationship. On the contrary, it is crucial for the newborn to find confirmation that the other is able to comprehend and recognize a personal demand for human relationship, and physical and affective presence. (Mirror neurons are triggered in some behaviors but probably they are not the cause of these behaviors or the related emotions). Obviously the infant cannot use verbal language but is able to feel. The infant is extremely sensible to any kind of affections such as love, hate, coldness and is at the same time able to react to them. If the adult gives love and affection, adequately responding to the newborn's needs, it will undergo healthy growth. In addition, the infant will develop a safe attachment or in other words, it won't be afraid of being abandoned because its affective expectations have not been disappointed. Therefore the infant will gradually

separate from the mother during weaning, developing little by little its own autonomy. This process occurs together with verbal language development which should be considered as an infant personal and creative realization. According to this vision, the newborn is not a wax table on which to impress mental, cognitive or social abilities. During the developmental phases, every step forward will be firstly the outcome of a creative ability of the individual that happens along with neurofunctional maturation of the corresponding body system. If the newborn's needs and requirements have been satisfied during the first months of life together with an unconscious elaboration of the experience had during breastfeeding, this will increase vitality. This will lead the infant to an ever-increasing research of another human being during its growth. The infant will become more confident acquiring an awareness of its and others identity. All these stages will lead the infant to the crucial stage of weaning. This is a fundamental stage of human development after birth and the first year of life without verbal language. In the past, the definitive end of maternal breastfeeding coincided with the beginning of deambulation and verbal language. (Until not many years ago, in Italy and also other countries breastfeeding continued beyond the first year of life due to a lack of nourishment and an approximate birth control). Nowadays food weaning usually ends within the first 7–8 months of life. By saying this, we more widely intend the time in which the infant begins to become more independent from adults. In fact, during this stage the baby starts speaking and walking. If the newborn has had healthy relationships until this moment, he/she will have acquired a personal certainty and comprehension of the human world, along with the abilities that allow to be relatively independent. In this situation the infant will realize a complete separation of oneself from the other significant adult. In other words, the baby will not experience anguish. From a psychodynamic point of view, weaning will physiologically occur after having satisfied one's desire for the substance of the other. For further reading, see [8]. During the 8th–9th months infants have developed a certainty of their identity which will allow them to recognize their face in the mirror. This will happen even if they have never seen themselves before, causing a reaction of joy at the vision of their face.

6. Pathology

The capability of being well with oneself and others, being an active part of society is fundamentally influenced by the first year of life. If the infant's demand for love and acceptance is constantly disappointed due to relationship that aims only at addressing physical needs, the infant will suffer an unsatisfactory experience. The internal elaboration won't develop a sense of trust or well-being but rather a feeling of insecurity and struggle between a natural tendency toward others and the constant disappointing answer received. In these conditions, the original vitality will be compromised. After going through stages of rage and progressive loss of vitality, an alteration in the relationship characterized by pathological dynamic of introjection and projective identification will occur. On this point, we suggest reading Chapter 2 in [1] and Chapter 4 in [7]. Although altered, these dynamics will still allow a relation with human reality. If in the early stages no other valid human relationship occurs to change this condition, there will be a further evolution toward pathology. The child, in order to defend oneself from the external aggressive human reality, altered by dynamics of introjective and projective identification will annul the existent human world. In other words the infant will make mentally disappear the disappointing human reality. By doing so, personal humanity and capability to love will disappear too. The annulment pulsion, without vitality, will be addressed toward the human reality, perceived as inanimate, and consequently as non-human. This is a physiological pulsion at birth, as it is turned toward non human reality such as light. Moreover, at birth this pulsion has in itself vitality. Now it is pathological: firstly because of its lack of vitality and secondly because it is addressed toward humans. We recommend the first three books of Massimo Fagioli for a complete explanation of what has just been briefly synthetized [1, 7, 8]. The dynamic explained can occur in the earliest months of life and will determine the onset of serious mental pathology such as schizophrenia in the most serious cases. The signs of this illness will appear only years later. Regarding this pathology we must consider both hebephrenic and simplex schizophrenia, erased in DSM V. The former is identifiable as disorganized and undifferentiated in the DSM-IV-TR whereas the latter not any longer considered, does not comprehend altered behaviors for a long time, sometimes the whole life, if not only with social withdrawal which we still consider a serious mental illness (Bleuler provided a clear specification of the symptoms of these clinical pictures, [28]). In other cases, mental illness can occur later during the first year of life or at weaning with the onset of other serious mental illnesses such as different forms of schizophrenia (paranoid and catatonic to maintain a reference to classic nosography) and depression which is still more likely to be successfully treated. The core of pathology is the formation of *anaffettività* that addresses the annulment pulsion toward humans, decreasing the individual own libidinal abilities [1, 16]. In the most serious condition the subject makes disappear the whole or part of the human reality of the other because unable to establish a rapport. This dynamic will be triggered not only toward disappointing beings but this mechanism will appear in any human relationship that might be significant or able to touch our deepest dimension. If nobody intervenes to contrast this non conscious relation, the individual will annul every possibility to establish a deep relationship, by making the human world meaningless, and consequently impoverishing its own identity. The core of mental illness finds its roots in the non-conscious individual internal reality. Behavior, language, symptoms and evident signs of pathology must be considered as a direct consequence. The basic dynamic is the annulment pulsion against the human reality. In a nutshell, we can consider two pathological mechanisms that reinforce each other: the annulment pulsion against human and the deficiency—loss of vitality—that leads to an increasing impoverishment of one's humanity and capability to feel the other (this can be partially identified with empathy, although it is wider concept). In this way, lack of affection (*anaffettività*) of another human being or another caregiver in touch with the newborn can turn into an infant or adolescent anaffective dimension which will usually manifest itself during adolescence or in the earliest stages of adulthood. (In a more or less extensive way from schizophrenic to schizoid to serious depression or other personality disorders such as narcissistic and borderline). A clear reconstruction of the pathological cycle can be found in [16]. I would like to reassert that anaffectivity connected with the annulment pulsion is related to human reality. In regards to material or external reality, adults can develop a sense of indifference and defense, which is not pathological. Moreover this theory helps to comprehend how much mental pathology and its non-conscious reality might be hidden in an apparent behavioral normality.

7. Psychotherapy

How can the Theory of Birth be applied to the psychotherapeutic treatment? The psychodynamic psychotherapy drawn from this Theory is based on some fundamental principles: a lack of affection in early human relationships can determine the onset of mental illness. At the same time, it is also true that mental illness can be cured through the therapeutic relationship with a healthy therapist who does not present a split between conscious and unconscious dimensions. Obviously this treatment must be based on a medical and clinical method, allowing the therapist to elaborate a psychodynamic diagnosis and prognosis. These have to be constantly verified and monitored throughout the treatment in order to propose a cure for recovery. According to this theoretical approach and clinical practice, psychotherapy is conceived as a medical act that aims at deeply modifying the individual's non-conscious reality. The therapist must be able to refuse the patient's non-conscious violent dimensions. This refusal can occur by identifying and contrasting these realities and by being able to respond to the request of being cured, which even in ambiguous way is a patient's demand. The annulment pulsion and negation are the two fundamental pathological dynamics that the psychotherapy, based on the Theory of Birth, aims at treating and curing. Both of them are non-conscious dynamics. (I shall recall that this psychotherapy mainly addresses the non-conscious mind whereas consciousness and behavior are considered as related to the internal reality). It has already been mentioned how the central core of mental pathology lies in the annulment pulsion which is split from vitality and it is addressed toward another human reality. The annulment pulsion annuls the human reality of the other. As a consequence, the subject itself realizes an emptiness which in turns annuls the possibility of any valid human relationship. This dynamic is strongly associated with many forms of schizophrenia, psychotic manifestation and manic excitement and to some extent to depression. It is also found in some personality disorders and in apparently normal people without evident behavioral disorders. Another common dynamic is negation, in which the subject perceives the other's psychic qualities (beauty, intelligence, sensibility, and interest for others) and immediately ruins, devalues or reverses them. This dynamic happens not so much consciously—in that case it should be considered as a lie—but rather in the non-conscious dimension by manifesting itself through dreams. For instance dreaming as ugly, deformed or stupid a person that in reality is not is a form of negation. Both the annulment pulsion and negation cause illness in human beings as they can result in damaging behaviors or conditions in which there is a lack or absence of interest for the other. A relevant example is the negation of human female qualities. This belief leads to the idea of female inferiority with tangible and dramatic daily consequences everywhere. The annulment of the human reality of another human being can lead to consider this as an object with devastating effects on the individual. In the most dramatic situations we have seen humans becoming object of trafficking, slavery and trade. However, this annulment can be modulated in such a way that it does not always give rise to physically violent behaviors. An example is given by adults that consider only children's physical needs during their growth and not their demand to establish a rapport and being recognized for their identity. This annulment pulsion has major effects on the children's psyche and body. Both the annulment pulsion and negation can determine malaise or the onset of mental illness. However, both cause the pathogenesis of illnesses in the subject acting these same dynamics: the annulment pulsion against human reality makes the subject itself 'anaffettivo' (lacking in affection); the negation of one's or others' qualities makes the individual depressed or envious. In the psychotherapeutic process based on the Theory of Birth, dreams interpretation is crucial to make a diagnosis. Non-conscious human thought expresses itself through oniric images during the night. This originates from the capability to imagine at birth and it is connected to the first year of life. In these images current psychopathological conditions manifest themselves. This point drastically differs from other classical psychoanalytic conceptions and in particular the Freudian one, according to which there is no major difference between hallucinations and dreams. These are considered as incoherent daily remnant or 'satisfaction of desire' [29]. According to the psychotherapy based on Theory of Birth, the diagnosis is always a dynamic process and must be related to the personal moment that the patient is experiencing. As it is susceptible to changes and modifications, it should be considered neither as a label nor as a conviction. In the psychotherapeutic relation proposed by Massimo Fagioli with its clinical method, the therapist becomes the object of a relationship with someone who seeks cure. In this relationship the patient will manifest all the unhealthy dynamics that affect his/her personal life. The therapist's interest is particularly focused on the interhuman conscious and non-conscious relationship that arises during the setting. 'Frustrating' unhealthy dynamics is a tool for the cure. In other words, it is fundamental for the therapist to verbalize and pretend that the patient sees and comprehends these dynamics. Only in this way the patient will become able to refuse them, by making them disappear. The patient can achieve this by finding in the relationship with the therapist the vitality that he/she had previously lost in unhealthy relationships. The patient will find that 'disappearance fantasy' experienced at birth and will become able to address this toward those unhealthy interior dimensions. In this rapport, it is crucial that the patient realizes a separation from those relationships that impedes a more profound change. In contrast with what happens in the everyday life, the therapist can interpret and frustrate these dynamics. Moreover, the therapist who was previously cured cannot be confused or attacked by these violent dimensions because of his/her personal vitality and creativity. In this sense the patient does not have the power to think of being omnipotently able to destroy the other. By doing so the patient avoids experiencing a sense of emptiness connected with the annulment pulsion. Furthermore, the therapeutic relationship addresses negative feelings, reducing the suicidal risks and self-destructiveness of depressed patients. The patient starts realizing that it is stimulating and beneficial to maintain a relationship with someone who is not psychically violent. In the case of psychotic patients, it can be crucial for them to experience the constant presence and interest of a human being that proposes a valid human relationship. Another fundamental point in the therapeutic work is the conceptualization of a 'hurtful absence' and the critic of the therapist's absence. For further references we suggest Chapter 1 in [1]. A major point is also the idea that the patient is active in the psychotherapeutic work. Facing another human being who has not lost its original identity and is able to realize a separation from another human relationship without annulment or negation is a crucial realization for the patient. This dynamic encourages the patient to understand and investigate how this could possibly occur. On a wider scale, this dynamic also happened in the Analisi Collettiva's experience. A brief and effective story of this phenomenon and its cultural implications can be found in a writing by Massimo Fagioli [30]. This method is used in much smaller groups and also in individual psychotherapy by many psychiatrists and psychotherapists that in addition to an academic formation in psychiatry and psychology have followed this story and experience firstly as patients.

8. Conclusion

In this chapter the physiology and pathology of the mind have been discussed according to the Theory of Birth by Massimo Fagioli. A particular attention was given to the following topics: the moment of birth, the mind physiological development and the onset of mental illness. Three are the most fundamental concepts. Firstly we must clearly define the dynamics of human birth physiology in which the newborn biological reality, by 'coming to light' immediately creates a merged non-conscious mental reality. Secondly, mental illnesses are an acquired condition affecting the irrational non-conscious dimension which main cause is to be found in social and human disappointing relationships lacking in affection. Lastly, it is possible to pursue a psychotherapeutic treatment based on this theory. This psychotherapy is based on a conscious and non-conscious therapeutic relationship between a healthy human being—the therapist who offers his/her own mental health and human reality as well as professional skills—and one who becomes ill because of a deficiency of conscious and non-conscious affection in human relationships. In particular this is a medical act, which has the intent to cure. Furthermore the physiology of birth is a dynamic equal for all human beings. Consequently the dynamics arising from it are universal. The Human Birth Theory constitutes a solid theoretical apparatus which has had significant effects on mental health care activities and has huge implications not only on the anthropological view of man itself and the ideas concerning its nature and human sociality, but also on bioethics [31]. Thanks to the Human Birth Theory, the unconscious is not unknowable or unmodifiable any more: non-conscious reality is a fundamental part of human reality which can be known and function in harmony with consciousness and, if altered, can be cured.

Author details

Irene Calesini
Mental Health Center, Local Healthcare Authority, Monterotondo, Rome, Italy

*Address all correspondence to: iri.cale@gmail.com

References

[1] Fagioli M. Istinto di morte e conoscenza. 14th ed. Roma: L'Asino d'oro edizioni; 2017. 345 p. ISBN: 978-88-6443-015-7 (German translation: Todestriebe und Erkenntis. Frankfurt am Main und Basel: Stroemfeld Verlag; 2011. 270 p. ISBN: 978-3-86600-076-6)

[2] Fagioli M. Bambino donna e trasformazione dell'uomo. Roma: L'Asino d'oro edizioni; 2013. 341 p. ISBN: 978-88-6443-004-1

[3] Dario M, Del Missier G, Stocco E, Testa L. L'istituzione rifiutata. In: Dario M, Del Missier G, Stocco E, Testa L, editors. Psichiatria e psicoterapia in Italia dall'unità ad oggi. Roma: L'Asino d'oro edizioni; 2016. pp. 597-609. ISBN: 978-88-6443-341-7

[4] Fagioli M. Materia Energia Pensiero. Roma: L'Asino d'oro edizioni; 2016. 272 p. ISBN: 978-88-6443-014-0

[5] Fagioli M. Conoscenza dell'istinto di morte. Roma: L'Asino d'oro edizioni; 2017. 247 p. ISBN: 978-88-6443-016-4

[6] Fagioli M. Left 2014. Roma: L'Asino d'oro edizioni; 2017. 301 p. ISBN: 978-88-6443-033-1

[7] Fagioli M. La Marionetta e il burattino. Roma: L'Asino d'oro edizioni; 2011. 322 p. ISBN: 978-88-6443-002-7

[8] Fagioli M. Teoria della nascita e castrazione umana. Roma: L'Asino d'oro edizioni; 2012. 307 p. ISBN: 978-88-6443-003-4

[9] Hevner RF. Development of connections in the human visual system during fetal mid-gestation: A Dil-tracing study. Journal Neuropathology and Experimental Neurology. 2000;**59**: 385-392. DOI: 10.1093/jnen/59.5.385

[10] Dubois J, Kostovic I, Judas M. Development of structural and functional connectivity. In: Toga AW, editor. Brain Mapping: An Encyclopedic Reference. Vol. 2. Amsterdam: Academic Press, Elsevier; 2015. pp. 423-437. DOI: 10.1016/B978-0-12-397025-1.00360-2

[11] Gatti MG, Becucci E, Fargnoli F, Fagioli M, Adén U, Buonocore G. Functional maturation of neocortex: A base of viability. Journal of Maternal-Fetal and Neonatal Medicine. 2012;**25** (S1):101-103. DOI: 10.3109/14767058.2012.664351

[12] Judas M, Sedmak G, Kostovic I. The significance of the subplate for evolution and developmental plasticity of the human brain. Frontiers Human Neuroscience. 2013;7(article 423):1-9. DOI: 10.3389/fnhum.2013.00423

[13] Kostovic I, Jovanov-Milosevic N. The development of cerebral connections during the first 20–45 weeks' gestation. Seminars in Fetal & Neonatal Medicine. 2006;**11**:415-422. DOI: 10.1016/j.siny.2006.07.001

[14] Vanhatalo S, Kaila K. Development of neonatal EEG activity: From phenomenology to physiology. Seminars in Fetal & Neonatal Medicine. 2006;**11**: 471-478. DOI: 10.1016/j.siny.2006.07.008

[15] Sernagor E, Young C, Eglen SJ. Developmental modulation of retinal wave dynamics: Shedding light on the GABA saga. Journal of Neuroscience. 2003;**23**:7621-7629. DOI: 10.1523/JNEUROSCI.23-20-07621.2003

[16] Maccari S, Polese D, Reynaert ML, Amici T, Morley-Fletcher S, Fagioli F. Early-life experiences and the development of adult diseases with a focus on mental illness: The human birth theory. Neuroscience. 2017;**342**: 232-251. DOI: 10.1016/j.neuroscience.2016.05.042

[17] Fagioli M. Capacità di reagire. In: Fagioli M, editor. Left 2011. Roma: L'Asino d'oro edizioni; 2014. pp. 231-235. ISBN: 978-88-6443-030-0

[18] Tinsley JN, Molodtsov MI, Prevedel R, Wartmann D, Espigulé-Pons J, Lauwers M, et al. Direct detection of single photon by humans. Nature Communications. 2016;7:12172. DOI: 10.1038/ncomms12172

[19] Polli D, Altoè P, Weingart O, Spillane KM, Manzoni C, Brida D, et al. Conical intersection dynamics of the primary photoisomerization event in vision. Nature. 2010;**467**(7314): 440-443. DOI: 10.1038/nature09346

[20] Gatti MG. Leggere la biologia e la vita umana [internet]. 2008. Available from: https://vimeo.com/30130265 (from 1 h to 1.05')

[21] Fagioli M. Vorstellungsvermögen. In: Fagioli M, editor. Left 2006. Roma: L'Asino d'oro edizioni; 2009. pp. 148-151. ISBN: 978-88-6443-025-6

[22] Fagioli M. Die Vorstellung. In: Fagioli M, editor. Left 2011. Roma: L'Asino d'oro edizioni; 2014. pp. 69-73. ISBN: 978-88-6443-030-0

[23] Freud S. In: Freud S, editor. OpereTre saggi sulla teoria sessuale. Vol. 4. Torino: Bollati Boringhieri; 1989. pp. 443-546. ISBN: 88-339-0474-1

[24] Stern D. Le prime relazioni sociali: il bambino e la madre. Roma: Sovera Multimedia; 1989. 195 p. ISBN: 88-85119-23-9

[25] Murray L. Le prime relazioni del bambino. Milano: Raffaello Cortina; 2015. 270 p. ISBN: 9788860307507

[26] Beebe B, Lachmann FM. Le origini dell'attaccamento. Milano: Raffaello Cortina; 2015. 337 p. ISBN: 9788860307637

[27] Spitz RA. Il primo anno di vita del bambino. Firenze: Giunti; 2009. 160 p. ISBN: 9788809742499

[28] Bleuler E. Dementia praecox o il gruppo delle schizofrenie. Roma: Carocci; 1985. 366 p. ISBN: 8843006266

[29] Freud S. L'interpretazione dei sogni. In: Freud S, editor. Opere. Vol. 3. Torino: Bollati Boringhieri; 1989. pp. 121-130. ISBN: 88-339-0473-3

[30] Fagioli M. La psichiatria come psicoterapia. Il sogno della farfalla. 2013; **4**:9-80 (PsycINFO)

[31] Calesini I. Fagioli's human birth theory and the possibility to cure mental illness. International Journal of Environment and Health. 2017;**8**: 185-192. DOI: 10.1504/ IJENVH.2017.086188

Chapter 3

Assessing Quality of Life in Children and Adolescents Diagnosed with Pulmonary Tuberculosis

Dinara Adjablaeva

Abstract

Work is devoted to studying the quality of life parameters of children and adolescents with different forms of tuberculosis. Laboratory and instrumental methods of examination of patients do not cover all aspects of tuberculous infection and do not allow valuing the condition of children and adolescents with pulmonary tuberculosis. During the analysis of quality of life parameters, there is a possibility to define the influence of the disease on physical, psychological, and social aspects of the organism's functioning. The analysis of quantitative indexes children and adolescents quality of life was conducted depending on gender sign, area of residence, and form of tuberculosis. For research of quality of life in pediatric practice, the questionnaire of Pediatric Quality of Life Inventory—PedsQL—is used. The questionnaire of PedsQL 4.0. includes 23 questions, incorporated in 4 scales. Every question has 5 variants of answers: "no," "hardly ever," "sometimes," "often," and "almost always," from which one has to be chosen, most going near a situation.

Keywords: quality of life, analysis, children, adolescents, tuberculosis

1. Introduction

The World Health Organization (WHO) estimated that nearly one third of the population of the planet is infected with *Mycobacterium tuberculosis* (MBT), as 8–10 million new active cases of pulmonary tuberculosis (TB) are registered annually [1]. The general epidemic situation on tuberculosis for the last 10–15 years has negatively affected the incidence of tuberculosis in children. First, the contact with adults suffering from tuberculosis, especially with bacterial isolation, causes new cases of infection of MBT in children. At the same time, social and economic reforms have given to considerable decrease in number of healthy children in structure of younger generation – from 4 to 10% [2]. In modern social and economic conditions, a relevant task is to create optimum conditions for healthy motherhood, providing the birth and development of a healthy child [3, 4]. Becomes obvious that negative processes of formation of health of younger generation are connected with growth of socially caused diseases at children and pregnant women, in particular tuberculosis [5]. The development of health care has put in the forefront the need for assessing the health of a child taking into account many, first of all social, factors [6]. During an economic crisis, the leading value, from the point of view of maintaining health, is on the quality of life of the child and his or her family members [7]. In recent years, the directions of studying the quality of life of children in clinical and in social pediatrics have extended [8]. WHO has suggested considering quality of life (life quality) as an optimum condition of perception by certain people and the population in general how their requirements as opportunities for achievement of well-being and self-realization are given are satisfied. Tuberculosis, influencing the physical state and psychology of behavior of an individual, changes his or her place and role in society [1]. In this regard, one of the new criteria for the evaluation of efficiency of delivery of health care is the quality of life. Today, it sounds as follows: the quality of life is a perception by an individual of his or her situation in life in the context of culture and the system of values in which the individual lives, and in connection with the purposes, expectations, standards, and the interests of this individual [9]. As quite often health depends on the level of availability of medical care, WHO considers the general availability of medical care of acceptable quality to children and adolescents mandatory at the present stage of development of society. Traditional criteria do not cover all aspects of a tuberculosis infection and do not allow estimating a condition of the sick child comprehensively. During the analysis of the quality of life parameters, there is an opportunity to define the influence of a disease on physical, psychological, and social aspects of functioning of an organism [10]. The use of this simple and reliable method will allow to improve the quality of medical care at different stages of treatment to children with chronic diseases, in particular, TB patients.

2. Purpose

To carry out the analysis of initial level of quality of life at children and adolescents depending on a sex, age, when using various methods of detection of a disease, to estimate indicators of quality of life depending on a form of tubercular process.

3. Materials and methods

In the conditions of children's department of the Samarkand State tuberculosis hospital, 90 children and adolescents aged 5–18 years subdivided into various subgroups have been examined. The quality of life was estimated by gender (2 subgroups: girls—56 and boys—34) and in various age groups (3 subgroups: adolescents aged 13–18 years—27 persons, children of school age 8–12 years—44 persons, children of preschool and younger school age 5–7 years—19 persons). Pulmonary tuberculosis has been for the first time revealed by means of various techniques: during inspection of risk groups by means of the medicine Diaskintest, the digital fluorographic device "ProScan 2000" was used as a recourse for medical care. The surveyed are divided into 3 relevant subgroups of 30 children and adolescents. For a century around the world, tuberculin was used for the diagnosis of tuberculosis and the detection of the latent tuberculosis infection. The main lack of tuberculin test is the large number of false positive reactions, in connection with cross-reactions of the antigens, which are contained in many species of mycobacterium and in strains of a bacillus of Calmette-Guerin (BCG). Diaskintest® (allergen recombinant in standard cultivation) is the recombinant protein produced by genetically modified culture of *Escherichia coli* and contains two antigens (ESAT-6 and CFP-10) that are present at virulent strains of mycobacterium of tuberculosis and absent in a vaccinal strain of BCG. With an intradermal injection of Diaskintest® for persons with a tuberculosis infection, a specific skin reaction, which is a delayed-type hypersensitivity, develops. This reaction is absent in people vaccinated with BCG and not infected with MBT. Because of the outbreaks of tuberculosis that have become frequent around the world, in recent years, the value of fluorography as an identification method has increased. The main advantages of digital photofluorography are high informational content of the image, the minimum dose at inspection, convenience of archiving and extraction of data, lack of an X-ray film and chemicals, and high bandwidth of the equipment. The digital fluorography became comparable with survey radiographic pictures. It means that the ability to detect the pathology sharply increases during mass inspections. Dose loadings from the simplest digital photofluorography are 10 times less. Such small dose allows expanding the age group for X-ray prevention of tuberculosis. At the same time infiltrates and the centers come to light with big constancy in all departments of lungs and have the outlined borders; disintegration cavities, come to light always convincingly; lymph nodes distinctly are found in zones, inaccessible to an ordinary radiological research. If necessary it is possible to send pictures for expeditious consultations on computer networks, and the consultant not the subjective report of the surveying doctor, and primary diagnostic information is transferred to any distances.

In terms of the clinical forms, the primary forms of tuberculosis prevailed in 50 (55.6%) patients: tuberculosis of intrathoracic lymph nodes in 34 (37.8%) patients and primary tuberculosis complex in 16 (17.8%). The secondary forms of tuberculosis prevailed in 40 (44.4%) respondents: tuberculous pleurisy in 3 (3.3%), disseminated tuberculosis in 12 (13.3%), and infiltrative tuberculosis in 25 (27.8%) patients. On the basis of these forms, patients have been divided into two subgroups.

In all subgroups, the analysis of initial level of quality of life was carried out. For a research on quality of life in pediatric practice, the questionnaire of Pediatric Quality of Life Inventory—PedsQL— proved effective. For the assessment of quality of life, all 23 criteria have been united in 6 scales: FF—physical functioning, EF—emotional functioning, SF—social functioning, SF—life in a school/garden, PSF—psychosocial functioning, and TS—a total scale. Answers to these questions open such problems for the child as the ability for independent movement and active actions, the self-service level, the emergence of pain and also experience of negative emotions, sleep disorder, and difficulties in communication with peers, problems in training, etc. The questionnaire is divided into blocks depending on age—5,–7, 8–12, and 13–18 years. The total of points pays off on a 100-mark scale after the procedure of scaling: the total size is higher, the quality of life of the child is better. Answers of children were expressed further in points. In the questionnaire for children of 5–7 years, 3 possible answers in connection with age features of these children were offered, and the graphic system of answers was used: the symbolical image of the person with a smile meaning "never," persons with the neutral expression meaning "sometimes," and persons with the negative expression meaning "often." For children of 8–12 years and adolescents of 13–18 years, each question has 5 possible answers: "no," "almost never," "sometimes," "often," and "almost always," from which it is necessary to choose one, the most suitable to a situation. All children answering the questionnaire had no mental disease according to the basic and associated diseases. Statistical processing of results of the research was carried out with the use of Microsoft Excel 2007 programs. Quantitative signs are presented in the form of average arithmetic ± a standard mistake. The statistical analysis was carried out by means of a statistical package of the SPSS program (Statistical Package for the Social Sciences Inc., USA) version 14.0 in Russian. The analysis of data included standard methods of descriptive and analytical statistics. The t-test for independent selections, t-test for dependent selections, and the one-factorial dispersive analysis (ANOVA) were used for the comparison of average values of selections. Correlation analysis was applied to establish communication between parameters of quality of life and social factors. The probability of a mistake $p < 0.05$ was regarded as significant, $p < 0.01$—very significant, and $p < 0.001$—the most significant.

4. Results

4.1 Quality of life of patients depending on gender sign

The comparative analysis of initial level of quality of life separately on gender sign has not revealed significant differences on a total scale—61.7 ± 2.3 and 59.4 ± 3.5 points (**Table 1**). However, subjective indicators of physical functioning for boys were much higher, than those for girls—66.5 ± 2.3 and 56.2 ± 3.5 points. Boys noted difficulties in lifting heavy objects by registering feeling of pain in extremities and low level of energy more often. It is more difficult for girls to cope with physical activities in the form of a run or a long walk; they noted weakness and difficulty in performing daily household activities more often. On the scale of emotional functioning, indicators are higher for girls—65.8 ± 3.9, than those for boys—61.2 ± 3.3 points, and they have revealed the high level of viability to new conditions; however, existence of such problems as emotional sensitivity and internal dissatisfaction with the appearance of a chronic disease is noted. In boys, emotional problems are generally connected with sleep disorders and feeling of aggression and rage because of the state of and need for a long hospital stay and also existence of fear, uncertainty in the future. Points on the scale of social functioning for boys are also authentically higher, than those for girls—62.1 ± 3.7 and 50.1 ± 2.9 that is explained by aspiration of boys to leading and self-realization in children's and adolescents collective. The main problem points noted by boys were connected to impossibility to quickly improve the relations with peers. Girls often pointed that peers often teased them, and it was difficult to feel on an equal basis with healthy children. At the same time, difficulties when performing tasks in school led to a considerable decrease in an indicator and school functioning of boys, than girls—56.7 ± 2.5 and 65.8 ± 2.4 points. For girls, difficulties with storing and concentration were observed more, and they skipped classes in connection with feeling sick more often. Nevertheless, in the analysis of a total scale of psychosocial functioning, indicators have appeared low, but are higher for boys (61.4 ± 3.6) than for girls (58.9 ± 2.9).

4.2 Quality of life of patients depending on age

The analysis of quality of life in various age groups has shown that by criterion of physical functioning the highest rates are noted in subgroup of children of 5–7 years—60.2 ± 4.4 points (**Table 2**). As a rule, these children have only certain

Aspects of quality of life	Boys on = 34 (M ± σ)	Girls n = 56 (M ± σ)
Physical functioning	66.5 ± 2.3	56.2 ± 3.5
Emotional functioning	61.2 ± 3.3	65.8 ± 3.9
Social functioning	62.1 ± 3.7	50.1 ± 2.9
School functioning	56.7 ± 2.5	65.8 ± 2.4
Psychosocial functioning	61.4 ± 3.6	58.9 ± 2.9
Total scale	61.7 ± 2.3	59.4 ± 3.5

Table 1.
Indicators of quality of life of patients depending on gender sign (in points).

Aspects of quality of life	5–7 years n = 19 (M ± σ)	8–12 years n = 44 (M ± σ)	13–18 years n = 27 (M ± σ)
Physical functioning	60.2 ± 4.4	43.0 ± 3.0	52.6 ± 3.3
Emotional functioning	57.6 ± 5.2	48.3 ± 3.0	50.1 ± 3.2
Social functioning	58.3 ± 6.7	48.2 ± 3.1	40.2 ± 4.0
School functioning	39.2 ± 5.2	45.6 ± 2.0	48.9 ± 2.4
Psychosocial functioning	52.0 ± 4.5	47.3 ± 2.7	46.4 ± 3.0
Total scale	55.0 ± 4.4	47.8 ± 2.6	48.6 ± 3v2

Table 2.
Indicators of quality of life of patients depending on age (in points).

difficulties in performing household chores and lifting heavy objects, and a part of children noted fast development of fatigue. Indicators for children of 8–12 years were the lowest—43.0 ± 3.0 points, and they pointed to difficulties in performing physical activity at school and in the visited sport sections. It is explained by decrease in number and volume of physical exercises, restriction of participation in sports, and need for restraint during physical activities. In the subgroup of adolescents of 13–18 years, indicators of physical functioning were 52.6 ± 3.3 points, and these patients often pointed to difficulties in overcoming big distances on foot and when running, pain in various parts of the body, and lack of force. On the scale of emotional functioning, high rates also belong to children of 5–7 years—57.6 ± 5.2 points, and they often pointed to existence of a bad dream and depression of mood in connection with violation of a habitual day regimen. Similar indicators were approximately equal in the second and third subgroups of patients—48.3 ± 3.0 and 50.1 ± 3.2 points. Respondents often noted fear for the future, and some adolescents aggressively behaved that is caused by high knowledge of the disease and thereof emotional reaction of children of advanced age and adolescents. On the scale of social functioning, children of 5–7 years have the highest rates—58.3 ± 6.7 points, and they noted difficulties in the period of initial communication with the children who are, as well as themselves, in an antituberculous hospital. Children of 8–12 years pointed that, according to them, other children did not want to be on friendly terms with them and often teased them that has found the reflection on indicators of quality of life in social aspect—48.2 ± 3.1 points. In adolescents of 13–18 years, the lowest indicators on this scale—40.2 ± 4.0 points—are noted, and they noted the lameness in comparison with healthy age-mates—development of stigmatization in consciousness of adolescents. The scale indicator "school functioning" has authentically reflected the presence of social and psychological problems of children of the first subgroup suffering from tuberculosis—39.2 ± 5.2 points. At the age of 5–7 years, children begin to study at school, and there is a change of friends, collective, the mode; information loading that is a stress source. In view of the fact that during this period there was both an inspection and treatment of children concerning a tuberculosis infection; all this, certainly, was expressed in low indicators of school functioning. Children of 8–12 years and adolescents had higher rates on this scale of functioning—45.6 ± 2.0 and 48.9 ± 2.4 points. These subgroups of patients often skipped classes in connection with weight of the state and also had difficulties in storing of material, which has been presented to their attention. On the total scale of psychosocial functioning, indicators of all subgroups were close to each other, with small advantage in the first subgroup—52.0 ± 4.5, 47.3 ± 2.7, and 46.4 ± 3.0 points. From the results of the total scale of functioning, indicators of patients of the first group prevailed over the others—55.0 ± 4.4, 47.8 ± 2.6, and 48.6 ± 3.2 that testifies to high adaptation opportunities of children of younger school age.

4.3 Quality of life of patients depending on the disease form

Indicators of quality of life in groups of patients depending on the form of a disease are presented in **Table 3**.

The indicator of quality of life considerably differed at various methods of detection of tuberculosis of respiratory organs. On the scale of physical functioning, the highest rates are recorded in the first subgroup—revealed during inspection with the Diaskintest—65.4 ± 3.7— and it were patients who have been examined because of identification in family of the adult patient with active tuberculosis. These children and adolescents kept the physical functioning; only in a small part of children, some decrease in physical activity owing to existence of burdening due to the main disease pathology was noted. In subgroup of the patients revealed actively—at recourse for a medical care, indicators of quality of life in aspect of physical functioning the lowest indicators—55.1 ± 3.1 were that has been connected by existence of extensive process in a pulmonary parenchyma. These children and adolescents often observed bed rest and have been limited to activity within medical office. The subgroup of patients revealed by indicators of a physical state by digital fluorography was equal to average assessment on the scale of a physical state among all examined patients—60.9 ± 2.2 points (on average 60.5 ± 3.4 points). It demonstrates that the method of digital fluorography has revealed patients both with limited, and with pathology, widespread in a lung, which is reflected in different degree on their physical functioning. Indicators of emotional functioning of the patients revealed by the Diaskintest and digital fluorography have close and rather high rates—68.1 ± 2.8 and 65.1 ± 3.9 points. In these subgroups of patients, the existence of depression of mood owing to being diagnosed with a chronic disease was noted, many expressed concern about preservation of vigorous activity in the future. Indicators of social functioning of the patients revealed by the Diaskintest and digital fluorography also have rather high rates—71.4 ± 4.7 and 70.5 ± 3.2 points. At the same time at representatives of the third subgroup—the patients revealed at recourse for a medical care, to a thicket at adolescents with common and destructive forms of tuberculosis, authentically low results—54.9 ± 3.3 points are observed. In the patients of the third subgroup, the main reasons for decline in quality of life in the social sphere are they had restrictions in communicating with peers because of understanding of the infectious nature of the disease and their possible transmissibility for people around. Life at school for children and adolescents revealed by a test method with the Diaskintest and digital fluorography is broken to a lesser extent (64.8 ± 2.5 and 60.7 ± 1.5 points), than at identification at recourse for a medical care—54.7 ± 2.9 points. An average value on the scale of school functioning among all three subgroups surveyed was 60.1 ± 3.6 points.

Aspects of quality of life	Diaskintest	Digital fluorography	Recourse for a medical care	All
Physical functioning	65.4 ± 3.7	60.9 ± 2.2	55.1 ± 3.1	60.5 ± 3.4
Emotional functioning	68.1 ± 2.8	65.1 ± 3.9	47.2 ± 3.1	60.1 ± 3.7
Social functioning	71.4 ± 4.7	70.5 ± 3.2	54.9 ± 3.3	65.6 ± 3.1
School functioning	64.8 ± 2.5	60.7 ± 1.5	54.7 ± 2.9	60.1 ± 3.6
Psychosocial functioning	70.1 ± 4.4	68.4 ± 2.6	50.7 ± 2.8	63.1 ± 2.8
Total scale	68 ± 3.7	65.1 ± 3.1	52.5 ± 3.1	61.9 ± 3.3

Table 3.
Indicators of quality of life of patients depending on the method of identification (in points).

The received results speak about existence of problems in school, which are often connected with poor progress in such disciplines as mathematics, physics, and chemistry demanding bigger concentration and assiduity. The scale of psychosocial functioning as a result of scales of emotional and social activity has revealed big differences for the children and adolescents revealed at test with the Diaskintest—70.1 ± 4.4 points and at recourse for a medical care—50.7 ± 2.8 points that once again is confirmed by results on each of these scales. The average level of quality of life (a total scale) was the lowest at identification at recourse for a medical care—52.5 ± 3.1 points, the highest—children when carrying out have tests with the Diaskintest and carrying out digital fluorography in groups of the increased risk (68.0 ± 3.7 and 65.1 ± 3.1 points). The general point among all contingent surveyed was on average 61.9 ± 3.3 points.

4.4 Quality of life of patients depending on associated diseases

Indicators of quality of life in groups of patients depending on the form of disease are presented in **Table 4**.

Initial level of quality of life separately in forms of a disease has revealed insignificant distinctions on a total scale—63.7 ± 2.8 points—in the group of patients with primary forms of tuberculosis of respiratory organs and 59.9 ± 2.7 points for children and adolescents with secondary forms of a disease. However, subjective indicators of physical functioning for patients with primary forms were much higher, than in the second subgroup (67.5 ± 2.1 and 58.2 ± 3.4). It proves that the inflammatory process in respiratory organs is more extensive, it is more difficult for the patient to cope with physical activities in the form of a run or a long walk, and they noted weakness and difficulty in performance of daily household chores more often. Also for children and adolescents with secondary forms of tuberculosis, decrease in number and volume of physical exercises is noted. Indicators of emotional functioning are approximately equal in the first and second subgroup of patients—63.2 ± 3.7 and 64.8 ± 3.7 that reflect negative influences of a disease on an emotional condition of the patient regardless of the form of tuberculosis of respiratory organs. Children of both subgroups are emotionally unbalanced that is expressed in capriciousness, unwillingness for a long hospital stay, and refusal of medical and diagnostic manipulations. Social functioning in the group of children and adolescents with primary forms of tuberculosis is reliable above similar indicators in the second subgroup—64.7 ± 2.8 and 51.9 ± 2.4. This results from the fact that the general condition of patients of the first subgroup clinically does not change considerably; these forms of tuberculosis proceed most often with symptoms that do not influence communication with peers in a group, whereas secondary forms of tuberculosis in children and, especially, in adolescents proceed as clinically expressed that causes the necessity of temporary restriction of the

Aspects of quality of life	Primary forms n = 50 (M ± σ)	Secondary forms n = 40 (M ± σ)
Physical functioning	67.5 ± 2.1	58.2 ± 3.4
Emotional functioning	63.2 ± 3.7	64.8 ± 3.7
Social functioning	64.7 ± 2.8	51.9 ± 2.4
School functioning	51.7 ± 2.9	53.8 ± 1.8
Psychosocial functioning	64.2 ± 2.6	56.3 ± 2.1
Total scale	63.7 ± 2.8	59.9 ± 2.7

Table 4.
Indicators of quality of life of patients depending on the form of disease (in points).

social activity by patients. So, adolescents of the second subgroup, patients with disseminate forms of tuberculosis, are forced to observe a high bed rest that, along with emotional depression, leads to narrowing of communication by other patients within the chamber or with the persons who are looking after them. On the scale of school functioning of reliable differences, it is almost not established—51.7 ± 2.9 and 53.8 ± 1.8 points. Patients, both in the first and second subgroups, equally often experience difficulties when performing tasks at school and skip classes because of feeling sick or needing medical manipulations. The scale of psychosocial functioning as total scale of emotional and social functioning has revealed authentically high rates of quality of life in the first subgroup of patients, than in the second—64.2 ± 2.6 and 56.3 ± 2.1. It is explained by the existence of numerous and ineffective courses of treatment of the anamnesis and by alarm and fear of uncertainty of the future. Children and adolescents of the second subgroup have big degree of consciousness and knowledge of the chronic pathology and realize the need for a continuous intake of medicines in the hospital conditions. It leads to lower indicators of quality of their life in comparison with patients of the first subgroup.

5. Conclusions

1. Influence of a chronic disease on quality of life of children and adolescents had gender specifics: in girls, it was the physical well-being, while for boys, more relevant were problems with functioning in school, first of all.

2. The estimated quality of life for children of 8–12 years and adolescents of 13–18 years is much below than for children of 5–7 years.

3. In group of the children revealed at recourse for medical care indicators of quality of life is lower, than on average among all surveyed.

4. Inspection methods are more extensive and more invasive, especially when decline in quality of life is experienced. According to priority diagnostics on the basis of test with the medicine Diaskintest in comparison with diagnostics at recourse for a medical care is.

5. Secondary forms of tuberculosis, widespread, with existence of destructive changes more influence indicators of physical and social functioning that is also reflected in total scales. The clinical form of the disease significantly does not influence indicators of emotional and school functioning of children and adolescents suffering from tuberculosis in respiratory organs.

Author details

Dinara Adjablaeva
Samarkand State Medical Institute, Samarkand, Uzbekistan

*Address all correspondence to: dinarasammi@mail.ru

References

[1] Zar HJ, Udwadia ZF. Advances in tuberculosis 2011-2012. Thorax. 2013;**68**(3):283-287

[2] Vinyarskaya IV, Rams AA, Albitsky VY, et al. Results, tasks and the prospects of studying of quality of life in domestic pediatrics. Questions of Modern Pediatrics. 2015;**3**:6-8

[3] Yuryev VK, Saifullin MH. Assessment of dynamics of quality of life of children as criterion of efficiency of hospitalization. Questions of Modern Pediatrics. 2012;**6**:7-11

[4] Solokhina LV, Dyachenko OA, Yarinchuk EI. Studying of quality of life of children, TB patients. Far East Medical Journal. 2016;**1**:134-137

[5] Osipova MA, Lozovskaya ME, Suslova GA. Quality of life at the children infected and TB patients, at a stage of sanatorium rehabilitation. News of the Samara Scientific Center of the Russian Academy of Sciences. 2015;**17**(5-3):844-848

[6] World Health Organization. WHO Report. 2017

[7] Perez-Velez C. Diagnostic of intrathoracic tuberculosis in children. In: Starke JR, Donald PR, editors. Handbook of Child and Adolescents Tuberculosis. New York: Oxford University Press; 2016. pp. 147-176

[8] Varni JW, Sherman SA, Burwinkle TM. The PedsQL™ Family impact model: Preliminary reliability and validity. Health and Quality of Life Outcomes. 2004;**2**:55

[9] Brown J, Cappoci S, Smith C, Morris S, Abubakar I, Lipman M. Health status and quality of life in tuberculosis. International Journal of Infectious Diseases. 2015;**32**:68-75. DOI: 10.1016/j.ijid.2014.12.045

[10] Gorbach L. Incidence rates of tuberculosis among children and adolescents living in areas most affected by the chernobyl disaster. Journal of Health and Pollution. 2016;**6**(10):28-41

Chapter 4

Ethanol

Kenechukwu C. Onyekwelu

Abstract

Ethanol with the molecular formula C_2H_6O is a clear, colorless, volatile liquid with a pleasant smell made by fermentation of sugar. Ethanol is one of many kinds of alcohol and is the only type of alcohol that can be consumed. Apart from consumption, ethanol is used for several other purposes such as fuel to power engines, as a disinfectant (because of its bactericidal activity), as a solvent and preservative as well as serving as the primary ingredient in the preparation of alcoholic beverages. In this chapter, the author describes how ethanol is metabolized in the body, genetics behind ethanol metabolism, metabolic pathways and hosts for ethanol production, ethanol and malnutrition, why ethanol is considered as a drug and effect of ethanol on neurotransmitter [gamma-amino-butyric acid (GABA), glutamate, dopamine, and serotonin] systems. The author further explains the effect of ethanol on antidiuretic hormone (vasopressin).

Keywords: ethanol, neurotransmitters, antidiuretic hormone, GABA, glutamate, dopamine, serotonin, metabolism

1. Introduction

Ethanol is a mood-altering drug with both pleasant and unpleasant effects. It is a clear liquid that is made by the fermentation of different biological materials. Ethanol (CH_3CH_2OH) is an alcohol, a group of chemical compounds whose molecules contain a hydroxyl group, –OH, bonded to a carbon atom [1]. When an alcoholic beverage is consumed, it passes through the stomach into the small intestine where it is rapidly absorbed and distributed throughout the body. Alcohol cannot be stored in the body and therefore, the body must metabolize it to get rid of it. It can only be metabolized in the liver, where enzymes are found to initiate the process. Ethanol is metabolized in the body to provide energy and does not have any minerals, vitamins, carbohydrates, fats or protein associated with it and as a result of this, it directly contributes to malnutrition. General malnutrition is often reflected in body weight loss, mainly of adipose and muscle tissue. This loss of nutritional reserves is partly due to inadequate protein intake in the face of continued alcohol ingestion. Alcohol is very rich in energy, packing seven calories per gram. The more calories an individual consumes in alcohol, the less likely it is that the individual will eat enough food to obtain adequate nutrients. More ethanol is found in the blood and the brain than in muscle or fat tissue. Alcohol acts as a central nervous system (CNS) depressant and as a diuretic and affects several neurotransmitter systems within the brain such as glutamate, gamma-amino-butyric acid (GABA), dopamine and serotonin systems. Ethanol is also used as a fuel for internal combustion engines either alone or in combination with other fuels and has both short and long-term economic advantages over fossil fuel. One striking advantage of ethanol over other fuel sources is that it does not cause pollution to the environment thereby reducing global warming which is caused by relentless emission of dangerous greenhouse gases emanation from use of fossil fuels.

2. Metabolism of alcohol

When an alcoholic beverage is consumed, it passes through the stomach into the small intestine where the ethanol is rapidly absorbed and distributed throughout the body and more ethanol is found in the blood and the brain than in muscle or fat tissue. Around 2–8% of consumed alcohol is lost through urine, sweat, or the breath and the other 92–98% is metabolized in the liver. Alcohol is metabolized by several pathways. These pathways involves four enzymes—alcohol dehydrogenase (ADH), aldehyde dehydrogenase (ALDH), catalase and microsomal ethanol oxidizing system (MEOS). These enzymes help break apart the alcohol molecule, making it possible to eliminate it from the body. In the first step, the primary pathway for alcohol metabolism involves alcohol dehydrogenase (ADH), a cytosolic enzyme that catalyzes the conversion of alcohol to acetaldehyde, a highly toxic substance and known carcinogen [2] (**Figure 1**). ADH is found mainly in the liver but can also be found in other organs of the body such as brain and stomach. During the process of conversion of ethanol to acetaldehyde, ethanol binds to alcohol dehydrogenase enzyme and loses some of its electrons in the form of hydrogen atoms to a coenzyme nicotinamide adenine dinucleotide (NAD) to form NADH. Ethanol oxidation generates an excess of reducing equivalents in the liver, mainly as NADH. NADH participates in numerous metabolic reactions in the body and for proper functioning of the body; the ratio of NAD to NADH must be tightly controlled. The conversion of ethanol to acetaldehyde by alcohol dehydrogenase enzyme reduces the cellular NAD to NADH ratio and this has profound effects on other liver metabolic pathways that require NAD or are inhibited by NADH. Decreased NAD/NADH ratio inhibits important reactions in the body such as glycolysis, tricarboxylic acid cycle (TCA cycle), fatty acid oxidation, pyruvate

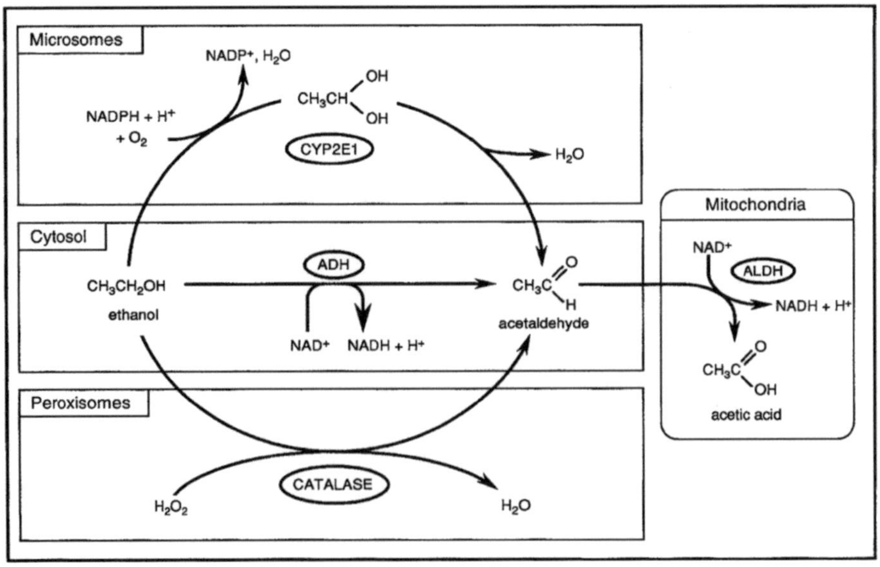

Figure 1.
Metabolism of ethanol to acetic acid/acetate.

dehydrogenase and gluconeogenesis. Altered NAD/NADH ratio/elevated cellular NADH levels may lead to several metabolic disorders. Elevated levels of NADH could lead to the formation of abnormally high levels of lactic acid, which in turn reduces the capacity of the kidney to excrete uric acid. Excessive uric acid in the body can lead to gout, a disorder characterized by extremely painful swelling of joints [3]. Increased NADH promotes the generation of the building blocks of fat molecules (fatty acids) and reduces the breakdown of fats in the liver, thereby contributing to fat accumulation in that organ [4]. The resulting fatty liver is the earliest stage and the most common form of alcohol-induced liver disease. The elevation in NADH levels resulting from the ADH-mediated breakdown of alcohol also may play a role in the formation of scar tissue that characterizes fibrosis, a more severe stage of liver disease.

Another pathway is the microsomal ethanol oxidizing system (MEOS). The primary component of the MEOS is the cytochrome P450, which exists in several variants. The variant most important for alcohol metabolism is cytochrome P450 2E1 (CYP2E1) [5]. This pathway uses NADPH as a coenzyme in the metabolism of ethanol and results in the formation of NADP and water (**Figure 1**). The cytochrome CYP2E1/MEOS pathway is only active after a person has consumed large amounts of alcohol [6]. Alcohol breakdown by microsomal ethanol oxidizing system generates several highly reactive oxygen-containing molecules called reactive oxygen species (ROS). These reactive oxygen species can damage liver cells by inactivating essential enzymes and altering the breakdown of fat molecules and when there is an imbalance between ROS and antioxidant systems, a condition known as oxidative stress sets in which can cause liver cell damage. Alcohol and its metabolism have been shown to reduce the levels of both glutathione (GSH) and vitamin E (α-tocopherol) which protects the body against ROS [6]. The catalase pathway metabolizes only a small fraction of alcohol in the body [2].

In the second step, acetaldehyde is further metabolized down by aldehyde dehydrogenase (ALDH) to another less active by product called acetate (**Figures 2** and **3**) which in turn is broken down into carbon dioxide and water. Ethanol is mainly eliminated from the body via metabolism into carbon dioxide and water. Acetate/acetic acid combine with Coenzyme A to form acetyl-CoA. The acetyl-CoA enters the tricarboxylic acid (TCA) cycle/Krebs cycle. In the Krebs cycle, acetate in the form of acetyl CoA is broken down into carbon dioxide and in this process ATP is formed (**Figure 3**) [2]. Some individuals have less effective forms of ethanol metabolizing enzymes and can experience more marked symptoms from ethanol consumption than others [7].

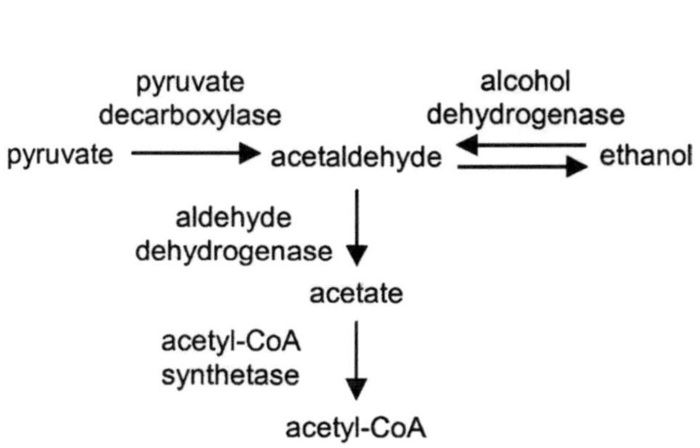

Figure 2.
Acetaldehyde dehydrogenases in ethanol and pyruvate metabolism.

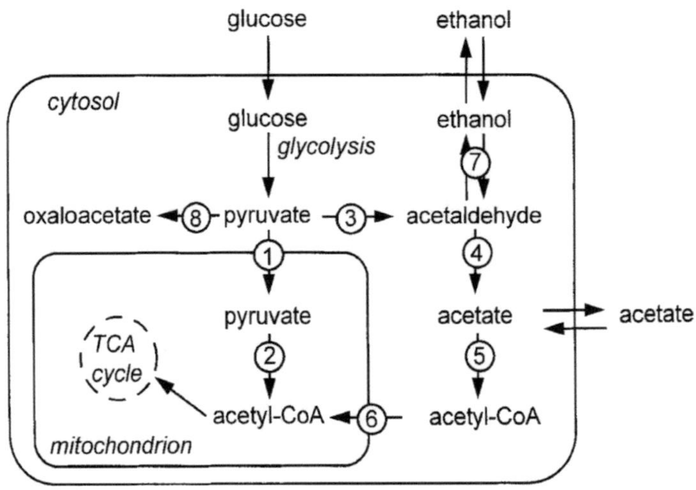

Figure 3.
Metabolism of ethanol to acetyl CoA. Numbered reactions are catalyzed by the following enzymes: 1: mitochondrial pyruvate carrier; 2: pyruvate dehydrogenase complex; 3: pyruvate decarboxylase; 4: acetaldehyde dehydrogenase; 5: acetyl-CoA synthetase; 6: carnitine shuttle; 7: alcohol dehydrogenase; 8: pyruvate carboxylase.

3. Genetics behind ethanol metabolism

Important factors that can influence responses to alcohol are variations in alcohol-metabolizing enzymes. Genetically influenced metabolic factors have been implicated in the etiology of alcoholism among different ethnic groups. Several genetically determined variants of ADH and ALDH enzymes exist that differ in their level of activity and different people have different variants of these enzymes. Some of these enzyme variants work more or less efficiently than others; this means that some people can break down ethanol to acetaldehyde, or acetaldehyde to acetate, more quickly than others. The type of ADH and ALDH an individual carries has been shown to influence how much he or she drinks, which in turn influences his or her risk for developing alcoholism [8].

Genetic differences in ADH and ALDH enzymes may help to explain why some ethnic groups have higher or lower rates of alcohol-related problems. There are multiple ADH and ALDH enzymes that are encoded by different genes. These genes occur in several variants and the enzymes encoded by these alleles can differ in the rate at which they metabolize ethanol or acetaldehyde or in the levels at which they are produced and these variants have been shown to influence a person's drinking levels and consequently the risk of developing alcohol abuse or dependence [8]. Studies have shown that people carrying certain ADH and ALDH alleles are at significantly reduced risk of becoming alcohol dependent. The mechanism through which ADH and ALDH variants influence alcoholism risk is thorough the elevation of acetaldehyde levels, resulting either from a more rapid ethanol oxidation or from slower acetaldehyde oxidation. Acetaldehyde is a toxic substance whose accumulation leads to a highly aversive reaction.

Humans have seven different ADH genes called ADH1A, ADH1B, ADH1C, ADH4, ADH5, ADH6, and ADH7 and there are three different ADH1B alleles: the ADH1B*1 allele, ADH1B*2 (this allele is common in Asians) and the ADH1B*3 (this allele primarily is found in people of African descent) alleles. The ADH1B*2 allele is associated with rapid ethanol oxidation and has shown protective effects against alcohol dependence in a variety of populations and ethnic groups. ADH1B*2 allele is found at high frequency in East Asians and it has been shown to be protective against alcoholism [8, 9]. ADH1B*2 allele is not very common in European or

African populations but also provides protection against alcoholism [10]. ADH1B*2 allele is found at moderate frequencies among people of Jewish descent and reduces binge drinking and risk for alcoholism [11, 12]. The protective effect of ADH1B*2 appears to be weaker in European than in Asian populations [10]. This difference could result from different social and environmental factors. The ADH1B*3 allele had a significant protective effect on risk for alcoholism in a set of African-American families selected for having multiple alcoholic members [13].

Numerous polymorphisms exist in the human ALDH genes, some of which cause inborn errors of metabolism and contribute to clinically relevant diseases [14]. Several isozymes of ALDH have been identified, but only the cytosolic ALDH1 and the mitochondrial ALDH2 metabolize acetaldehyde produced during ethanol oxidation [8, 15]. Polymorphism in the ALDH2 gene is associated with altered acetaldehyde metabolism, alcohol-induced 'flushing' syndrome, decreased risk for alcoholism and increased risk of ethanol-induced cancers. Genetic polymorphism of the ALDH2 gene result in allelic variants ALDH2*1 and ALDH2*2. ALDH2*2 allele is relatively common in people of Chinese, Japanese, and Korean descent but is essentially absent in people of European or African descent [8, 16]. People carrying an ALDH2*2 allele show an alcohol flush reaction, even when they consume only relatively small amounts of alcohol [17]. In these people, acetaldehyde levels in the blood increase from nearly undetectable levels to levels high enough to trigger the highly aversive reactions.

4. Metabolic pathways and hosts for ethanol production

Ethanol is produced from glucose via fermentative consumption of pyruvate, the end product of glycolysis [18]. Glycolysis is a metabolic process that converts glucose to pyruvate while producing ATP. The pyruvate formed by glycolysis is further metabolized via one of the three catabolic routes. In aerobic organisms or tissues, under aerobic conditions, pyruvate is oxidized with the loss of its carboxyl group as CO_2 to yield the acetyl-CoA; the acetyl-CoA is then completely oxidized to CO_2 in the citric acid cycle (**Figure 4**). The second route for pyruvate is its reduction to lactate via lactic acid fermentation in vigorously contracting muscle. Under anaerobic condition, pyruvate is reduced to lactate. Another major route of pyruvate catabolism leads to ethanol. In some plant tissues and certain invertebrates, protists and microorganisms such as brewer's yeast, pyruvate under anaerobic conditions can be fermented to ethanol by sequential reactions of pyruvate decarboxylase (PDC) and alcohol dehydrogenase (ADH) (**Figure 4**).

Microbial fermentation was introduced by Louis Pasteur in the late 1850s and was the first to recognize the relationship between the presence of yeast cells and the conversion of sugar to ethanol. Today ethanol producing *Saccharomyces cerevisiae* (yeast) have been exploited to produce a wide variety of alcoholic beverages and biofuels. Many microorganisms are being used for ethanol and biofuel production, but all have certain limitations such as industrial robustness, substrate utilization, productivity and yield. *Saccharomyces cerevisiae* (yeast) is a leading traditional industrial biocatalyst microorganism for ethanol production and with technological advancement in genetic engineering, bacteria such as *Escherichia coli*, *Zymomonas mobilis*, *Corynebacterium glutamicum* and *Bacillus subtilis* have been developed [19].

Zymomonas mobilis (*Z. mobilis*), a bacterium commonly found in plant saps and in honey has many desirable industrial biocatalyst characteristics and has been suggested as an alternative to the classical model, *Saccharomyces cerevisiae* (yeast) due to its advantage for ethanol yield. *Saccharomyces cerevisiae* uses the Embden-Meyerhof-Parnas (EMP) pathway for glycolysis while *Z. mobilis* uses the Entner-Doudoroff

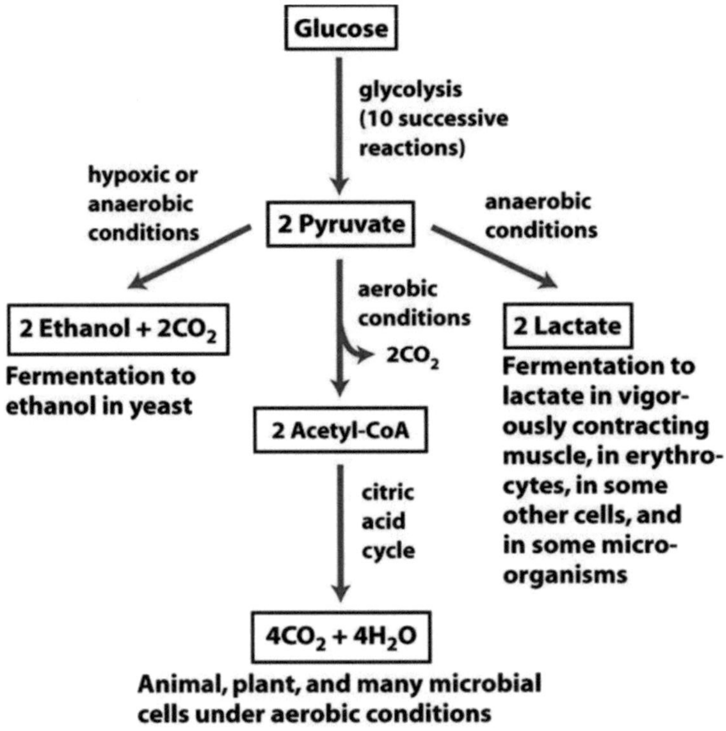

Figure 4.
Three possible catabolic fates of pyruvate formed in glycolysis (adapted from Lehninger principles of biochemistry).

(ED) pathway. The ED pathway is found in strict aerobic microorganisms and conducts fermentation with 50% less ATP produced relative to the EMP pathway, which leads to improved ethanol yield. Moreover, *Z. mobilis* has a high-specific cell surface area and consumes glucose faster than *S. cerevisiae*, leading to higher ethanol productivity than *S. cerevisiae* [20] (**Figure 5**). Although the EMP pathway is a major glycolytic route in most eukaryotes and prokaryotes, glycolytic pathways are much more diverse in prokaryotes [21]. Among different glycolytic pathways, the ED and EMP pathways are the most abundant pathway for glycolysis [21]. Two molecules of ATP are produced from each molecule of glucose consumed using EMP pathway, while the ED pathway produces only one ATP molecule from one glucose molecule. Given that ATP is tightly coupled with anabolism and cell growth, ED pathway-utilizing *Z. mobilis* produces less energy than EMP pathway-dependent species such as *S. cerevisiae* and consequently, *Z. mobilis* has more available carbons for ethanol fermentation with 2.5-fold higher specific ethanol productivity than that of *S. cerevisiae* [22].

Z. mobilis is an obligately fermentative bacterium which lacks a functional system for oxidative phosphorylation. Like the *Saccharomyces cerevisiae*, *Z. mobilis* produces ethanol and carbon dioxide as principal fermentation products. Ethanol is produced by *Z. mobilis* using a short pathway which requires two enzymatic activities: pyruvate decarboxylase and alcohol dehydrogenase. Pyruvate decarboxylase is the key enzyme in this pathway which diverts the flow of pyruvate to ethanol. In this pathway, the non-oxidative decarboxylation of pyruvate to produce acetaldehyde and carbon dioxide is catalyzed by pyruvate decarboxylase. In *Z. mobilis*, two alcohol dehydrogenase isozymes are present which catalyzes the reduction of acetaldehyde to ethanol during fermentation.

DOI: http://dx.doi.org/10.5772/intechopen.79861

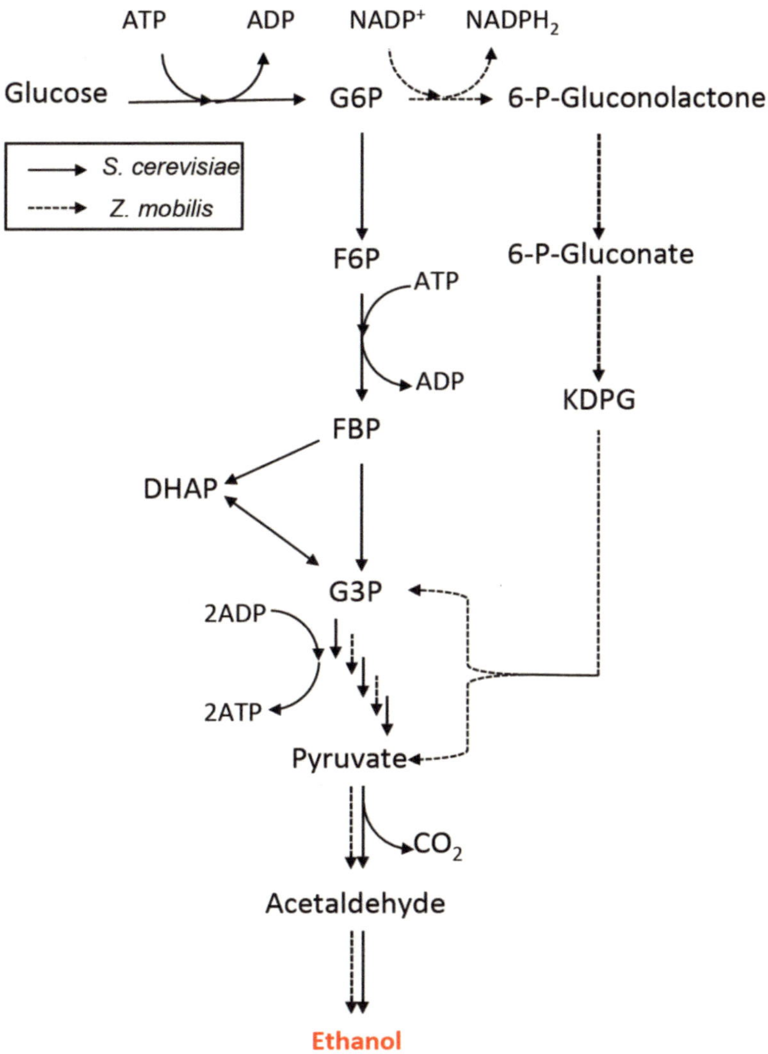

Figure 5.
Ethanol fermentation pathways in S. cerevisiae and Z. mobilis (solid line: EMP glycolysis pathway; dashed line: ED glycolysis pathway). KDPG: 2-keto-3-deoxy-6-phosphogluconate; G6P: glucose 6-phosphate; F6P: fructose 6-phosphate; FBP: fructose 1,6-bisphosphate; DHAP: dihydroxyacetone phosphate; G3P: glyceraldehyde 3-phosphate.

5. Ethanol and malnutrition

Ethanol consumption has an effect on person's nutritional status. Many people who consume one to two glasses or less of alcoholic beverages per day consider those beverages a part of their normal diet and acquire a certain number of calories from them. When consumed in excess, ethanol can interfere with the nutritional status of the consumer. Ethanol can alter the intake, absorption and utilization of various nutrients [23, 24]. The primary constituents of alcoholic beverages are water, ethanol (alcohol), sugars (carbohydrates) and negligible amounts of other nutrients like proteins, vitamins and minerals. Because alcoholic beverages provide almost no nutrients, they are considered as "empty calories". Any calories provided by alcoholic beverages are derived from the carbohydrates and alcohol they contain. Ethanol has a caloric value of 7.1 kcal/g.

Many consumers of alcoholic beverages suffer from various degrees of malnutrition (both primary and secondary malnutrition). A situation where alcohol replaces other nutrients in the diet resulting in overall reduced nutrient intake is known as primary malnutrition while secondary malnutrition occurs when alcoholics consumes adequate nutrients but alcohol interferes with the absorption of those nutrients from the intestine so they are not available to the body [25]. The risk of developing micro- and macronutrient deficiencies increases significantly when alcohol makes up more than 30% of total caloric intake [26]. Heavy alcohol consumption not only influences the drinker's diet but also affects the metabolism of those nutrients that are consumed. Even if the drinker ingests sufficient proteins, fats, vitamins, and minerals, deficiencies may develop if those nutrients are not adequately absorbed from the gastrointestinal tract into the blood, are not broken down properly, and/or are not used effectively by the body's cells.

Proteins are essential nutrients for the human body that help maintain the cell's structure, act as enzymes that mediate almost all biochemical processes/reactions occurring in the body and transport certain substances in the body. Amino acids are building blocks of proteins and proteins are composed of 20 different amino acids. Some of these amino acids can be made by the body itself (non-essential amino acids) from various precursors or are recycled when proteins that are damaged or are no longer needed are broken down or degraded. Other amino acids cannot be produced by the body and must be obtained through diet (essential amino acids). Heavy alcohol consumption can interfere with the production and uptake of these non-essential and essential amino acids. Vitamins are micronutrients present in food essential for normal metabolism and insufficient levels of vitamin in the body can lead to serious health consequences. Alcoholics tends to have deficiencies in certain vitamins particularly thiamine (vitamin B1), riboflavin (vitamin B2), pyridoxine (vitamin B6), ascorbic acid (vitamin C) and folic acid.

6. Ethanol as a psychoactive drug and its effect on neurotransmitters

Ethanol is a psychoactive substance which is present as the active ingredient in alcoholic beverages such as beer, wine, and distilled spirits [27]. Ethanol consumption produces mood lift and euphoria, decreased anxiety, increased sociability, sedation, impairment of cognitive, memory, motor, and sensory function, and slows down the activity (depressant) of the central nervous system (CNS) and because of its psychoactive effects, it is considered a drug. Psychoactive substances are those substances that act on the nervous system to alter states of consciousness, modify perceptions and change moods. Psychoactive drugs are classified into depressants, stimulants and hallucinogens. Depressants slow down physical and mental activity; Stimulants increases the activity of the central nervous system while Hallucinogens modify perceptions and produce unusual visual images.

Human behaviors and emotions are modulated by neurotransmitters that act as keys between neurons. Ethanol has been shown to affect a variety of neurotransmitters in the CNS. A neurotransmitter is a chemical that helps transmit messages from cell to cell within the nervous system and are crucial to muscle control, influences thought processes, memory and emotion. Alcohol mainly affects the nerve cells in the brain, causing interference between communication of these cells and other cells throughout the body. This interference restrains the activities of the excitatory nerve pathways and increases the activities of inhibitory nerve pathways. Alcohol affects several neurotransmitter systems—those for GABA, glutamate, serotonin and dopamine. Alcohol is an agonist for GABA, serotonin and dopamine—it increases their activity and is an antagonist for glutamate—it reduces glutamate activity.

Neurotransmitters interact with receptors on the dendrites of the other neuron and have specific shapes that fit into a receptor that can accommodate that shape. Once the neurotransmitter and the receptor are connected, the neurotransmitter sends information to the next neuron to either fire an action potential, or to inhibit firing (**Figure 6**). Neurotransmitters can either be excitatory or inhibitory according to the effect they have on the second neuron once they are released into the synaptic gap. Excitatory neurotransmitter triggers depolarization, increasing the likelihood of a response while inhibitory neurotransmitter triggers hyperpolarization, decreasing the likelihood of a response. Excitatory and inhibitory synaptic transmission use different neurotransmitters and receptors. Excitatory synaptic transmission uses a neurotransmitter called glutamate. Glutamate is a common amino acid used in the body to build proteins. In the central nervous system, it is the major excitatory neurotransmitter where it interacts with glutamate receptors in the post-synaptic neuron. These receptors are ion channels that are permeable to sodium ions (Na^+) and thus generate an action potential. Excitatory synaptic transmission also uses other neurotransmitter like acetylcholine, nitric oxide and catecholamines (norepinephrine, epinephrine and dopamine).

Inhibitory synaptic transmission uses a neurotransmitter called gamma-amino butyric acid (GABA). This interacts with GABA receptors, ion channels that are permeable to negatively charged chloride ions and opening of these channels makes it harder for a neuron to generate an action potential. Inhibitory synaptic transmission also uses serotonin, glycine and taurine as neurotransmitter. The main inhibitory neurotransmitter in the brain is GABA [28] and two major subtypes of GABA receptor have been described. The $GABA_A$ receptor family of ligand-gated ion channels consists of pentameric complexes containing binding sites for GABA agonists and other agent. The $GABA_A$ receptor complex regulates chloride ion flux through a coupled chloride channel and ethanol is widely reported to increase the activation of $GABA_A$ receptors.

Ethanol is an indirect GABA agonist and psychotropic depressant of the CNS [29]. This property is associated with the action of alcohol on different neurotransmitters, including the stimulation of gamma-amino butyric acid and the inhibition of glutamate, the main central excitatory neurotransmitter. Alcohol potentiates the effects of GABA by acting directly on its receptors, enhancing their inhibitory effect which includes sedation, loss of inhibitions and relaxation [30]. The mechanism

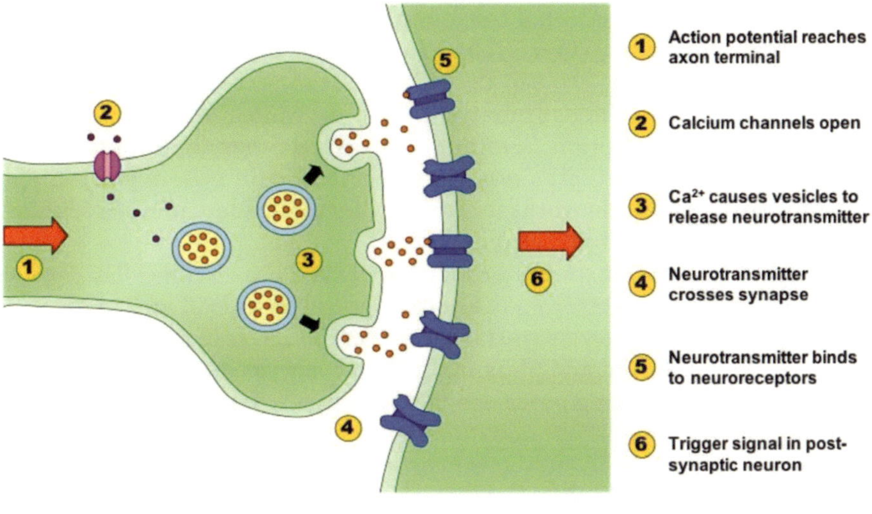

Figure 6.
Neuron-neuron interaction—transmission of impulse across the synapse.

by which ethanol enhances $GABA_A$ inhibitory currents involved a hyperpolarizing shift in the $GABA_A$ inhibitory postsynaptic current (IPSC) reversal potential in cortex neurons and increasing the amplitude of $GABA_A$ receptor-mediated conductance in septal neurons [31]. When $GABA_A$ receptor activation is enhanced by ethanol, it may involve enhancement of the initial peak of Cl^- current through the channel rather than the sustained component of channel opening [32]. The enhancement of the $GABA_A$ receptor activation by ethanol may be modulated, in part, by protein kinase C (PKC) [33].

Glutamate is a major excitatory neurotransmitter in the brain that exerts its effects through several receptor subtypes, including the N-methyl-D-aspartate (NMDA) receptor. Unlike the case with GABA, alcohol inhibits glutamate activity in the brain. In a region of the brain called striatum which contains the nucleus accumbens, ethanol exposure causes a drop in the extra cellular glutamate levels [34]. Following acute administration ethanol, glutamate mediated signal transmission is suppressed in the central nucleus of the amygdala and this effect is enhanced following chronic alcohol exposure [35]. Ethanol inhibits ionotropic glutamate, amino-3-hydroxy-5-methyl-4-isoxazole propionic acid (AMPA) and kainate receptors activity in the brain and N-methyl-D-aspartate (NMDA) receptors are the major target of ethanol's inhibitory action. Ethanol also inhibits the induction of neural plasticity in many brain regions including the dorsal and ventral striatum as a result of inhibitory effects on ionotropic receptors, especially the NMDA receptors [36, 37].

Serotonin is a monoamine neurotransmitter known as 5-HT, a derivative of tryptophan and is extensively found in the gastrointestinal tract, platelets and the CNS. Serotonin plays a role in many brain processes, including regulation of body temperature, sleep, mood, appetite, pain and modulates behavioral response to unfairness [38]. Defect with the serotonin pathway can cause obsessive-compulsive disorder, anxiety disorders and depression. Most of the drugs used to treat depression today work by increasing serotonin levels in the brain [39]. Alcohol increases serotonin release in the nervous system. Increase in concentrations of serotonin in the urine and blood have been observed after taking alcohol. Alcohol exposure alters various aspects of serotonin's synaptic functions and also interferes with the function of serotonin receptors including the $5\text{-}HT_{1A}$, $5\text{-}HT_{1B}$, $5\text{-}HT_2$, and $5\text{-}HT_3$ receptors. Each subtype of serotonin receptors has its own specific influence on behavior related to the consumption of alcohol [40]. $5\text{-}HT_{1A}$ may control consummatory behavior, including alcohol consumption while $5\text{-}HT_{1B}$ may contribute not only to alcohol's intoxicating effects, but also influence the development of tolerance to alcohol. $5\text{-}HT_2$ plays a role in alcohol's rewarding effects and contributes to the development of alcohol withdrawal symptoms while $5\text{-}HT_3$ has a part in regulating alcohol consumption. Serotonin also affects other neurotransmitters. For example, alcohol-facilitated serotonin may affect the GABA system [41]. Similarly, alcohol-influenced serotonin works to stimulate increased dopamine production and, thus, increased emotional behavior [42].

Dopamine is a neurotransmitter primarily involved in a circuit called the mesolimbic system, which projects from the brain's ventral tegmental area to the nucleus accumbens. It is an excitatory neurotransmitter in the catecholamine family responsible for modulating reward and pleasure. It plays a key role in regulating emotional responses, the reward seeking processes and movement. Several lines of evidence converge to demonstrate that the dopaminergic mesolimbic system plays a significant part in the motivational and reinforcement mechanisms related to behaviors that are vital to survival [43]. Alcohol increases dopaminergic transmission in the mesolimbic pathway and increases the firing rate of dopaminergic neurons, which enhances the amount of dopamine released in the core of the system.

7. Effect of ethanol on antidiuretic hormone (vasopressin)

Vasopressin is an antidiuretic hormone that plays a major role in the regulation of water excretion. The posterior pituitary gland releases vasopressin in response to a fall in blood volume or a rise in plasma osmolality and acts to conserve water by increasing the permeability of water to the distal convoluted tubules and collecting tubules in the renal nephrons through insertion of aquaporin-2 channels into the apical membrane of the tubular epithelial cells [44]. Ingestion of alcohol does increase plasma osmolality, but alcohol also acts directly to inhibit the release of vasopressin, independent of plasma osmolality. Once ethanol is consumed, it is distributed in the blood, brain and muscle tissues. Alcohol is a diuretic that affects five centers in the brain namely the cerebral cortex, limbic system, cerebellum, hypothalamus and pituitary gland and the medulla. The hypothalamus controls the automatic functions of the brain and coordinates endocrine functions through nerve impulse actions on the pituitary gland. Ethanol affects hypothalamus and pituitary gland by increasing urine excretion; inhibiting the pituitary secretion of anti-diuretic hormone (ADH), which makes the kidney reabsorb water. When the ADH levels are decreased, the kidney does not reabsorb water from the urine which results in the kidney producing more urine.

8. Conclusion

In conclusion, ethanol is a powerful drug that affects several neurological pathways such as the dopaminergic, serotoninergic, γ-amino butyric acid (GABA) and glutamate pathways and causes significant changes in the brain. It also affects the central nervous system and acts to depress brain functions, very much in the style of an anesthetic. Ethanol at low blood concentrations releases behaviors that are otherwise inhibited and usually produces feelings of relaxation and good mood which may facilitate socializing. Thus at low doses, ethanol is possibly useful but caution however needs to be exercised as even low quantities of alcohol affect the ability of the brain (hippocampus) to process information, which in turn impairs memory formation. Higher doses of alcohol affect the brain further by inducing intoxication wherein the person may experience temporary loss of coordination and judgment. Long-term alcohol abuse produces physiological changes in the brain and these changes in the brain chemistry maintain the alcoholic's compulsive inability to cease alcohol consumption being fully aware of the harm caused by alcohol and results in alcohol withdrawal syndrome upon discontinuation of alcohol.

Conflict of interest

I have no conflict of interest to declare.

Author details

Kenechukwu C. Onyekwelu
Department of Medical Biochemistry, College of Medicine, University of Nigeria, Enugu Campus, Enugu State, Nigeria

Address all correspondence to: kenechukwu.onyekwelu@unn.edu.ng

References

[1] National Center for Biotechnology Information. PubChem Compound Database; CID=702, https://pubchem.ncbi.nlm.nih.gov/compound/702 (accessed March 03, 2018)

[2] National Institute on Alcohol Abuse and Alcoholism. Alcohol Alert: Alcohol Metabolism. No. 35, PH 371. Bethesda, MD: The Institute; 1997 Available from: http://pubs.niaaa.nih.gov/publications/aa35.htm

[3] Lieber CS. Hepatic and other medical disorders of alcoholism: From pathogenesis to treatment. Journal of Studies on Alcohol. 1998;**59**:9-25

[4] Lieber CS, Schmid R. The effect of ethanol on fatty acid metabolism: Stimulation of hepatic fatty acid synthesis in vitro. Journal of Clinical Investigation. 1961;**40**:394-399

[5] Salmela KS, Kessova IG, Tsyrlov IB, Lieber CS. Respective roles of human cytochrome P-4502E1, 1A2 and 3A4 in the hepatic microsomal ethanol oxidizing system. Alcoholism: Clinical and Experimental Research. 1998;**22**:2125-2132

[6] Lieber CS. Relationships between nutrition, alcohol use, and liver disease. Alcohol Research & Health. 2003;**27**(3):220-231

[7] Agarwal DP, Goedde HW. Pharmacogenetics of alcohol metabolism and alcoholism. Pharmacogenetics. 1992;**2**(2):48-62

[8] Hurley TD, Edenberg HJ, Li TK. The pharmacogenomics of alcoholism. In: Pharmacogenomics: The Search for Individualized Therapies. Weinheim, Germany: Wiley-VCH; 2002. pp. 417-441

[9] Chen HJ, Tian H, Edenberg HJ. Natural haplotypes in the regulatory sequences affect human alcohol dehydrogenase 1C (ADH1C) gene expression. Human Mutation. 2005;**25**(2):150-155

[10] Whitefield JB. Alcohol dehydrogenase and alcohol dependence: Variation in genotype-associated risk between populations. American Journal of Human Genetics. 2002;**71**(5):1247-1250

[11] Luczak SE, Shea SH, Carr LG, Li T, Wall TL. Binge drinking in Jewish and non-Jewish white college students. Alcoholism: Clinical and Experimental Research. 2002;**26**(12):1773-1778

[12] Hasin ND, Aharonovich E, Liu X, Mamman Z, Matseoane K, Carr L, Li T. Alcohol and ADH2 in Israel: Ashkenazis, Sephardics, and recent Russian immigrants. American Journal of Psychiatry. 2002;**159**(8):1432-1434

[13] Edenberg HJ, Foroud T. The genetics of alcoholism: Identifying specific genes through family studies. Addiction Biology. 2006;**11**(3-4):386-396

[14] Vasiliou V, Pappa A. Polymorphisms of human aldehyde dehydrogenases. Consequences for drug metabolism and disease Pharmacology. 2000;**61**(3):192-198

[15] Crabb DW, Edenberg HJ, Bosron WF, Li TK. Genotypes for aldehyde dehydrogenase deficiency and alcohol sensitivity: The inactive ALDH2(2) allele is dominant. Journal of Clinical Investigation. 1989;**83**:314-316

[16] Oota H, Pakstis AJ, Bonne-Tamir B. The evolution and population genetics of the ALDH2 locus: Random genetic drift, selection, and low levels of recombination. Annals of Human Genetics. 2004;**68**(Pt. 2):93-109

[17] Peng GS, Yin JH, Wang MF, Lee JT, Hsu YD, Yin SJ. Alcohol sensitivity in Taiwanese men with different alcohol and aldehyde dehydrogenase genotypes. Journal of the Formosan Medical Association. 2002;**101**(11):769-774

[18] Ingram LO, Conway T, Clark DP, Sewell GW, Preston JF. Genetic engineering of ethanol production in *Escherichia coli*. Applied and Environmental Microbiology. 1987;**53**:2420-2425

[19] Dien BS, Cotta MA, Jeffries TW. Bacteria engineered for fuel ethanol production: Current status. Applied Microbiology and Biotechnology. 2003;**63**:258-266

[20] Conway T. The Entner-Doudoroff pathway: History, physiology and molecular biology. FEMS Microbiology Reviews. 1992;**9**:1-27

[21] Flamholz A, Noor E, Bar-Even A, Liebermeister W, Milo R. Glycolytic strategy as a tradeoff between energy yield and protein cost. Proceedings of the National Academy of Sciences of the United States of America. 2013;**110**:10039-10044

[22] Weber C, Farwick A, Benisch F, Brat D, Dietz H, Subtil T, Boles E. Trends and challenges in the microbial production of lignocellulosic bioalcohol fuels. Applied Microbiology and Biotechnology. 2010;**87**:1303-1315

[23] Lieber CS. Alcohol: Its metabolism and interaction with nutrients. Annual Review of Nutrition. 2000;**20**:395-430

[24] Lieber CS. Hepatic, metabolic and toxic effects of ethanol: 1991 update. Alcoholism: Clinical and Experimental Research. 1991;**15**:573-592

[25] Lieber CS. Alcohol-nutrition interactions. In: Li TK, Schenker S, Lumeng L, editors. Alcohol and Nutrition: Proceedings of a Workshop. Rockville, MD: National Institute on Alcohol Abuse and Alcoholism; 1979. pp. 47-63

[26] Tanaka Y, Funaki N, Mak IM, Kim C-I, Lieber CS. Effects of ethanol and hepatic vitamin A on the proliferation of lipocytes in regenerating rat liver. Journal of Hepatology. 1991;**12**:344-350

[27] Collins SE, Kirouac M. Alcohol consumption. Encyclopedia of Behavioral Medicine. 2013;**2013**:61-65

[28] Curtis DR. GABA synapses in the brain. Trends in Neurosciences. 1995;**18**:263

[29] Haes TM, Clé DV, Nunes TF, Roriz-Filho JS, Moriguti JC. Alcohol and central nervous system. Medicina (Ribeirão Preto). 2010;**43**(2):153-163

[30] Charlton ME, Sweetnan PM, Fitzgerald LW, Terwilliger RZ, Nestler EJ, Duman RS. Chronic ethanol administration regulates the expression of GABAA, receptor α 1 and α 5 subunit in the ventral tegmental area and hippocampus. Journal of Neurochemistry. 2002;**68**(1):121-127

[31] Soldo BL, Proctor WR, Dunwiddie TV. Ethanol differentially modulates GABAA receptor-mediated chloride currents in hippocampal, cortical, and septal neurons in rat brain slices. Synapse. 1994;**18**:94-103

[32] Nishio M, Narahashi T. Ethanol enhancement of GABA-activated chloride current in rat dorsal root ganglion neurons. Brain Research. 1990;**518**:283-286

[33] Weiner JL, Zhang L, Carlen PL. Potentiation of GABAA mediated synaptic current by ethanol in hippocampal CA1 neurons: Possible role of protein kinase CJ. Journal of Pharmacology and Experimental Therapeutics. 1994;**268**:1388-1395

[34] Carboni S, Isola R, Gessa GL, Rossetti ZL. Ethanol prevents the glutamate release induced by N-methyl-D-aspartate in the rat striatum. Neuroscience Letters. Mar 2, 1993;**152**(1-2):133-136

[35] Roberto M, Schweitzer P, Madamba SG, Stouffer DG, Parsons LH, Siggins GR. Acute and chronic ethanol alter glutamatergic transmission in rat central amygdala: An in vitro and in vivo analysis. The Journal of Neuroscience. Feb 18, 2004;**24**(7):1594-1603

[36] Lovinger DM, White G, Weight FF. Ethanol inhibits NMDA-activated ion current in hippocampal neurons. Science. Mar 31, 1989;**243**(4899):1721-1724

[37] Nie Z, Madamba SG, Siggins GR. Ethanol inhibits glutamatergic neurotransmission in nucleus accumbens neurons by multiple mechanisms. The Journal of Pharmacology and Experimental Therapeutics. 1994;**271**:1566-1573

[38] Crockett MJ, Clark L, Tabibnia G, Lieberman MD, Robbins TW. Serotonin modulates behavioral reactions to unfairness. Science. Jun 27, 2008;**320**(5884):1739

[39] Benmansour S, Cecchi M, Morilak DA, Gerhardt GA, Javors MA, Gould GG, Frazer A. Effects of chronic antidepressant treatments on serotonin transporter function, density, and mRNA level. The Journal of Neuroscience. 1999;**19**(23): 10494-10501

[40] Lovinger DM. The role of serotonin in alcohol's effects on the brain. Current Separations. 1999;**18**:23-28

[41] Samson HH, Harris RA. Neurobiology of alcohol abuse. Trends in Pharmacological Science. 1992;**13**:206-211

[42] Campbell AD, Kohl RR, McBride WJ. Serotonin-3 receptor and ethanolstimulated somatodendritic dopamine release. Alcohol. 1996;**13**:569-574

[43] Dulawa SC, Grandy DK, Low MJ, Paulus MP, Geyer MA. Dopamine D4 receptor-knock-out mice exhibit reduced exploration of novel stimuli. The Journal of Neuroscience. 1999;**19**:9550-9556

[44] Boone M, Deen PMT. Physiology and pathophysiology of the vasopressin-regulated renal water reabsorption. Pflügers Archiv. 2008;**456**:1005-1024

Chapter 5

Health Education and Lifestyles in the Czech Republic

Ludmila Fialova

Abstract

This chapter starts with the description of behavior, body care, health status, and demographic development in Europe, especially in the Czech Republic. It deals with the importance of physical activities for the whole population and with their benefits for self-concept, psychological and physical health, especially in the common time of sedentary life and increasing overweight and obesity. The author also introduces the new educational branch "Health Education" in the Czech Republic with the topics health support and prevention. The school subject health education integrates elements of the fields of sociology, psychology, medicine, and ethics. The aim is to educate the lifelong responsibility for own health, to build the positive inter-human relations, to create practical vitality and to support healthy social and mental life. Some habits as part of lifestyle in the Czech population and children's behavior are introduced in European comparison. Some research results illustrate lifestyles of common people and their typical characteristics of behavior, health care, their body image, and body care. The conclusions serve as recommendations for education in all ages in view of the weaknesses identified.

Keywords: psychological health, physical health, sedentary life, overweight, self-satisfaction, body care

1. Introduction

The lack of natural physical activity leads to growing masses of obese and ill individuals. On the other, we have seen a rise in eating disorders and other unfortunate practices that seriously damage the human body. There is no doubt that sufficient and appropriate physical activity should be included in lifestyles of people of all ages as it represents one of the most important factors of active and healthy aging [1–3].

Several sources report that children and youth spend the majority of their discretionary time engaging in sedentary activities (particularly watching television or playing video games) [4–7]. Engaging in regular physical activity is widely accepted as an effective preventative measure for a variety of health risk factors across all age, gender, ethnic, and socioeconomic subgroups [8–10].

Accumulating evidence shows that, independent of physical activity levels, sedentary behaviors are associated with increased risk of cardio-metabolic disease, all-cause mortality, and a variety of physiological and psychological problems [11–14]. Some studies deal with the relationship between sedentary behavior and health [15]. Most of them describe the relationship between screen time and body composition and do not include other indicators of health [16–18]. Regular physical activity reduced risks of cardiovascular disease, some types of cancer (e.g., breast and colon)

IntechOpen

and diabetes. It also helps to maintain the optimum body weight, improves the blood lipid profile, the digestive tract function, and mental health (reduces stress, increases self-esteem, and self-control and ability to concentrate) and boosts the body's immune system [19, 20]. Physical activity helps to control already existing health problems (e.g., diabetes, high blood pressure or high cholesterol levels), and it is important for maintaining physical, mental, and cognitive health in older age too. There is a link between physical activity and life expectancy, physically active people tend to live longer than inactive ones. On the other hand, insufficient physical activity, along with poor eating habits, leads to an increase in obesity in the population.

According to the report about the health of Czech citizens [21, 23], the most common causes of death in the Czech Republic in the long-term perspective is cardiovascular disease, kills 50% of the population. During the past 10 years, the mortality rate has been reduced by 20%, mainly due to the more effective diagnostic and therapeutic procedures. Compared to developed EU countries, the mortality rate due to the cardiovascular disease is twice as high in the Czech Republic. The mortality rate due to cancer is the second leading cause of death for both males and females in the Czech Republic. The incidence of new cases of the disease is steadily increasing, but the mortality rate remains at the same. In recent years, it has even been slightly declining. Severe disease with high-growth dynamics of morbidity includes diabetes mellitus. Allergic diseases represent a significant burden for public health and the economy. Asthma has become one of the most common chronic non-infectious diseases over the past few decades. Some habits of Czech population influence also health status. The use of tobacco products is among the most significant risk factors resulting in severe diseases and premature deaths, which can be effectively avoided by prevention. The number of smokers among adult citizens of the Czech Republic has been relatively stable in recent years, ranging between 28 and 32%. The Czech Republic has ranked first among all countries in the European region in the consumption of pure alcohol. High tolerance to alcohol consumption and using non-alcohol drugs, including cannabis, prevails in Czech society, especially among young people. Overweight and obesity present a major problem for a significant part of the Czech population. More than a half of the adult population in the Czech Republic (57%) has a higher than the standard weight and this proportion has not changed. Such a high proportion of the population in the overweight and obesity category is more characteristic of older men.

The total average number of healthy life years at birth in the Czech Republic was estimated at 62 years in 2010 [2]. This number is close to the EU average. Since 1962, however, this value has not changed. However, there are numerous countries where the situation is much more favorable. In Sweden, the time living in good health has increased by 9 years - up to 71 - over the same period, which is 9 years more than in the Czech Republic. The percentage of people who are not self-sufficient is increasing proportionally to age, with nearly 30% of people dependent on outside care found in the population of people over 80.

The aim of this chapter is to introduce the importance of lifestyle for human's health and his quality of life. We have the way of life in our hands (in contrast to heredity and some aspects of working/living conditions), and the recommended behavior can and should be supported by the government, education in schools, families, and other institutions, because there are many reserves and challenges for improvement. The submitted data are used from international comparative databases as EUROSTAT, COMPASS or from own research projects (the methodology is short explained in relevant chapters). This chapter is organized as follows. Section 2 describes the socioeconomic determinants and impacts to life; Section 3 portrays lifestyle in Czech Republic; next section presents results from previous empirical work, and finally, the conclusion is presented.

2. Socioeconomic determinants and impacts to life

We all are members of the same (materialistic) culture and have internalized in a certain way what is considered as important, wishful and worthwhile: that is, individual success, popularity, and financial prosperity. Living under external and often materialistic values may result in personal, social and ecological losses. On the personality level, consumption values may be related with lower personal well-being, lower frequency of pleasant emotional experiences in everyday life, a higher degree of depression, feeling of oppressiveness and narcissism, as well as it may be related with a higher probability for drug abuse and physical symptoms like head ache and stomach ache. Individuals who are more materialistically orientated take other people as an instrument for fulfilling their own interests. The ecological sphere gets hurt by a low interest of materialistic individuals concerning environmental protection and restoration of natural resources [26].

The present materialistic orientated culture proclaims the accumulation of property as the successful way. On the basis of the found search results, we can surely say that the individual well-being will not be increased by a new car or a villa on the sea.

2.1 Cultural changes

The status of people in society is based on their relations to the other people and results from experiencing the change in roles, lifestyle and economic security. This refers to transitioning into retirement, which represents a combination of several social changes: in the sphere of the role at work, the transformation of the parental role, a change in the relations between husband and wife, and a changed position in society.

The economic well-being of elderly people often limits them in their deeply rooted cultural and social activities. Besides, the socio-economic and health balance these people can further be affected by diseases, family problems, loneliness, the lack of finances, and poor housing. For this reason, people ought to be active until old age, participate in various social activities to maintain their social, mental, and physical balance as long as possible.

The demographics of aging is affected by the growth in the education and qualifications of the population, changes in the upbringing of children, changes in the lifestyle of the population and also the population migration from rural to urban areas.

The conditions of civilization are permanently more comfortable for human and demands on his condition are constantly lower, thanks to technological progress. In human development, the evolution process, more capable individuals got easier access to food, to reproduction opportunities, and physical abilities were source of authority. The biological evolution created human's body adapted to movement impulses for physical development, cultural evolution. On the contrary, it gives rise to a reduction of necessity of intensive physical effort. Nowadays, the human is in disharmony with the biological and cultural development. Its evolution inherited naturalness to prefer energetic valuable food (fatty and sweet) rather than to economize energy expenditure. Therefore, it results in positive energetic balance, obesity increase, bad condition and broadening lifestyle diseases.

The main blame for this situation is the substantial different lifestyle, which created a "*Homo sapiens*" in progress. Supporters of modernity correctly point out the fact that common human does not need the caveman's condition for his existence because he does not face to merciless prehistoric conditions (as hunger, coldness, and predators).

Summing up, there are differences in health-related behavior according to the historic moment considered, according to culture and its influence on perception and evaluation of human's body, on health oriented habits. Today society has enough information about health benefits of involvement in sports and its influences on desirable behavior and personal satisfaction. For this reason, institutions should support prevention of lifestyle diseases and active way of life.

2.2 Family education

The family life changed dramatically in the last years. Many parents do not have time enough for their children, for healthy cooking and common leisure activities. Parents and health authorities commonly view television and computers as barriers to physical activity, lack of time, environmental and cost factors and personal factors. Fear of strangers (12.4%) and lack of safe areas for children to play in within today's communities may limit opportunities and prevent the development of physical activity patterns at a young age. It may be far easier for children to stay inside with computers and television than to venture out into a dangerous neighborhood. An ecological perspective would, however, suggest that it is not sufficient to reduce television and computer time without providing spaces outside to play in, safe neighborhoods and low-cost activities. Thus a complicated myriad of factors is highlighted and all may require addressing in order to increase the level of children's physical activity.

Health authorities propose that increased physical activity is a primary factor in reducing overweight and obesity, and argue that participation in physical activity during childhood and adolescence increases the likelihood that activity is continued as an adult. Other benefits of physical activity include socialization and physiological and developmental factors. Watching television and playing computer games are two most common reasons for children not being more physically active.

In particular, girls in their teenage years may be at risk of increased societal and cultural pressures for women to be thin. In order to commence activities aimed at reducing weight, it is important that people perceive themselves or their children to have normal weight. There is no evidence of suggestion that adult perceptions of their children would be more accurate. Thus, if parents do not perceive their children as overweight, they are un-likely to encourage physical activity to reduce obesity or to address issues which may limit physical activity, such as dangerous neighborhoods and lack of space.

The majority of children's problems are solved instrumentally. The family ceases to be the example for children, emotional bonds loosen. The pace of life, interference of the media with all spheres of existence of man and pursuit of goods of consumption push realization of actual needs of children into the background. Poverty is more prevalent in families with single parents. Single parents, especially mothers and grandmothers have less time for their children in view of their job and duties in the household.

Home is the first setting where children have opportunities to foster an active life and motivate family members to be active. At home, children can practice and share what they learn about health and physical activity in the classroom. Parents, on the other hand, also hold important roles in the promotion of physical activity among children.

In summary, the active family life is very important. Parents are examples for their children in living healthy and having fun together. Working parents should believe that their investment to the common time with their children will help to both parent's and children's quality of life. Family is the most important institution in society, where children get first models for their behavior in the family. Eating habits and active participation in physical activity and sports influence the future behavior of children a lot. About 80% of obese children stay obese as adults not because of heredity, but because of habits. Family and parents play dominant roles in forming children's behaviors and habits also in physical activities. Children and adolescents are more likely to be physically active if their parents and siblings are also physically active. Parental support positively influences participation in sport among children and adolescents, and parents' attitudes toward physical activity can influence children's involvement in physical activity. Support of families with children and the offering of multiple leisure activities for families could be key to active and healthy people in the future.

2.3 School education

Physical activity programs offered by school are a platform, which can provide a bridge that links schools to their community. These opportunities allow involvement of volunteer organization, health care providers and representative of sports programs and other school to interact and enhance integration in the community. These social events are not only financially beneficial but is also creates awareness of the importance of physical activity in younger generation [30]. This collaboration can encourage better student behavior and social skills such teaching them responsible behavior in physical activity settings and the values of physical activity. Physical activity also creates a healthy understanding among students that school is not merely an academic platform to but also a place to access heath related fitness and to be competent in motor skills.

The new educational area focused on "Humans and health" in primary and secondary schools has been in place since 2007 in the Czech Republic. This educational area has been implemented in two subjects: Physical Education (practice) and Health Education (theory; either in one subject or inter-disciplinary).

Human health may be seen as a balanced state of physical, emotional, and social well-being. It is defined and influenced by several factors such as lifestyle, healthy conduct, interpersonal relationships, environment, and individual's safety and security. Health is a fundamental condition for guaranteeing a satisfying life and high work productivity. Learning about health, promoting health and preventing major health risks represent a priority of basic education [27].

Health Education gives pupils elemental knowledge about the perception, evaluation and preventative care of human body. Pupils learn active assistance and health cognizance of all its shapes (social, emotional, and physical) and responsibility for their own state of health. School leavers should be able to use their hygienic, eating, movement, work and other preventative healthcare habits, develop their power to decline harmful drugs, avoid trauma and deal with personal dangers in everyday and emergency situations. They develop and intensify their knowledge of family, peer group, society, nature, humans and interpersonal relationships, and learn to see their activities through the prism of the health-related needs and perspective of a growing young individual and to make decisions beneficial to the personal and also to the community health.

As part of pupils' comprehensive education in health-related Issues, the educational field of Physical Education focuses on becoming acquainted with one's personal abilities in physical activity and with the impacts of certain physical activities on physical fitness and emotional and social well-being. It starts with spontaneous physical activity and moves on to guided and elective activities aimed at giving pupils the ability to independently judge their level of physical fitness and to include physical activity into their daily routine, in order to promote the optimum development of fitness and performance, to recuperate strength and compensate for various forms of stress, and to promote health and health protection. The subjects include the knowledge of physical education (organization, practical order, hygiene, and safety), exercises for condition and compensation, motion games and main sports [28].

Adequate, regular and appropriate training should be provided by physical education or activity teachers. This may also be done by other staff members who may be responsible for motivating students for physical activities, such as health service staff, teachers of other subjects, and voluntary coaches. Not all countries have adequate resources and teachers providing Physical and Health Education.

Concluding, the school system should help to build expected and rational lifestyle. Pupils are motivated for activities if they learn them. Their attitudes are built the most in families and schools, and the cognitive component of attitude is key. We believe that emotion influences our attitudes; therefore, we have to create positive examples and experiences. The attitude is supported by specific practice, social communication, imitation/usual models, institutional factors, principal group, and culture. Health is the most important thing that we have Health Education in school is required, health oriented lessons could create systematic, deep and context knowledge.

3. Lifestyle in Czech Republic

Essential reality of the present is growth of own responsibility for actual state of individuals, for their own health state, fitness level, and of course lifestyle. The modern consumer lifestyle is characterized by overconsumption of different things and often by their wasting, by negligence to environment, by lack of physical activity, by excessive food consumption (often unhealthy), and drugs (alcohol, tobacco, medicine, and narcotics) abuse, by noise, hurry, disquiet, and mental overloading from impulses and information. It is a paradox that the human shortens his healthy life expectancy through excessive behaviors.

Disturbing is the fact that calling after healthier lifestyle is not new and recommendation for more emphasis on attention to healthier lifestyle, physical development and intentional effort for improvement of human's condition, are not successful enough. Movement tradition of Czech Falcon (Sokol) came into existence 160 years ago, modern mass sport also has 150 years old tradition and more than 100 years also has obligatory school physical education, which educates the whole population. The secondary school graduate went through approximately 1000 physical education lessons, where he learned what and why and how to exercise, and also he has a lot of voluntary opportunities to do sport in his leisure time. It has effects on some children who move with pleasure and enjoy social contacts during their physical activities too. Rational health education over the last 100 years has promoted incentives for development of skeletal muscular and heart pulmonary systems. Modern medicine produces undisputed research results that indicate that inactivity damages life systems and physical activity in daily regime supports health, life satisfaction and self-sufficiency. It is a paradox that everything mentioned above does not have a sufficient effect on physical activities in the human's life rather it decreases it. Startling is the fact that children and youth find amusement activities more in physically unambitious observation of virtual world of modern technologies, compared to a previous engagement in movement games. Body–mind imbalance in education is evident—not comparable greater attention is paid to opportunities for mental development than for physical advancement.

The task of all interventions through physical activity is to change sedentary behavior to active lifestyle. Adequate movement influences the human not only in biological but also in psycho-social aspects. It can so cultivate not only condition (fitness) and health state, but also integration to the society. It is deciding for regeneration after working and leisure loading area. Esthetically viewpoints help by struggle for condition. Since Antic time beauty believes are relatively constant. Actual discrepancy between ideal and statistical reality in population is rather large, for example, body mass index at attractive models is under 18, but a majority of self-compared women is nearly 10 points higher. The pressure on body treatment increases, not only through physical activities, but also through esthetic medicine and other through media promoted products.

Our health although depends on inborn factors, but it is possible to influence it by right regime – moderate nutrition, sufficiency of lifestyle, fresh air, mental balance, sleeping abundance, and hygiene.

3.1 Czech Republic lifestyle compared to some European countries

The active behavior as the part of lifestyle that influences the health and shows some important habits. We selected large and neighboring European countries for the presented comparison (Czech Republic, Finland, France, Germany, Poland, Austria, and Spain) [29].

Warning is the information about overweight and obesity in population aged 15 or over (according to Eurostat 2016). The highest overweight was founded in Czech females and males; pre-obesity is highest in Poland, and Czechs are on the second place, obese people are in the Czech Republic (but worse cases in Europe are Malta and Croatia). Not only objective, but also subjective well-being is determined by overweight and obesity [25].

Also, the distribution of smoking habits for the population aged 15 or over is warning. Most smokers are found in Poland (males) and Austria (females), but Czech Republic has the highest number of daily smokers (females and also males). Across all European countries, only people in Denmark smoke daily in the same rate as in Czech Republic.

The consumption of pure alcohol per capita in population 15 years and more harms the health too. The large number of consumers is found in France, Germany, and Austria; however, lately can be observed that Czechs are among the greatest drinkers (between all European countries drink more pure alcohol only people in Belgium and Austria).

Organized attendance in sports is satisfying in Youth, but very bad in adult population. In comparison to other, especially to the west and north European countries are Czechs adults significantly more passive as sport club members. They prefer unorganized forms of sport as walking, cycling, swimming alone or with friends irregularly in their leisure time. The most recent data on the participation in sports and physical activity has been provided by EUROBAROMETER 412 [21, 22]. This study found that, in EU, 48% of people participated in some type of physical activity at least once a week and 30% did not participate in any physical activity. The level of physical activity decreases with age—71% of men and 70% of women aged 55 or older participated in sports only rarely or never. Non-sporting physical activity may also improve people's lives and health. About 15% of EU citizens participate in a non-sporting physical activity (such as cycling, dancing, or gardening) 5 times or more per week. About one-third of EU citizens do these activities 1–4 times per week. About a half of EU citizens do not participate in this type of physical activity [21].

Also, cultural differences have been observed between various EU countries, above all between the Nordic countries and the rest. For example, 31% of Finnish and Swedish adults and only 6% of Bulgarian and Polish adults report that they participate in sports for health-related reasons. It is about 14% in the Czech Republic, which suggests that there is relatively low awareness of the importance of physical activity for health in the Czech adults. The situation of the Czech Republic can be illustrated further by the barriers the Czech adults mention in relation to their sporting physical activity. More than a half of them reported the lack of time as the most important barrier to physical activity. At the same time, in comparison with Nordic and other western countries, the Czech adults spent much more time sitting and watching TV [24].

As conclusion can be said that Czech Republic shows significant bad features concerning lifestyles, such as shortages in nutrition habits (all ages), lack in physical activities (older people), and love in cigarettes, alcohol and other drugs.

3.2 Children's habits and behavior

Children habits and lifestyles in Czech Republic are briefly described according to EUROSTAT (2016) [30]. Czech boys and girls prefer beer drinking before wine, but they drink spirits, wine, and beer more than their European peers (even though the law allows to pour alcohol in the restaurant to 18 old and older people only). There has been an increase of allergic children with larger incidence over boys than on girls in the Czech Republic. There is an increase of overweight between Czech population in age 15 years—boys (more) and girls and the number of overweight and obesity growths in all ages. We can see the type of participation in physical activities performed by young women and men (aged 11–18)—to the favorites belong competitive, organized and intensive activities and also irregular sporting in boys. Girls prefer no membership in sports club and irregular activities.

As a conclusion it may be inferred that lifestyles in Czech Republic do not tend to be healthy. Czech adults belong to the fattest European nations, they smoke and drink more than average and they participate in sports insufficiently. For this reason there is a large incidence of cardiovascular diseases. This may be considered as a warning to young people, because of the so-called in behavior. This behavior includes smoking, alcohol drinking, trying of drugs and playing computer games and other activities with smart phones and tablets (sedentary lifestyle) which are not favorable for health reasons. Czechs are very tolerant to different life ways, and the result is the long-term depraved life with misconducts against healthy life.

3.3 Lifestyles challenges

The growing technological, economic, cultural, biomedical, and social developments of European societies produce a high-level of comfortable living for a very large segment of population. For an increasing amount of inhabitants, the need to perform considerable physical activity in daily lives no longer exists. This results in a growing number of people who develop sedentary lifestyle. People today lead very different lives than their parents and grandparents did. For the most part, our generation is more educated, in better financial and geographical condition and more mobile than our predecessors.

It is generally accepted that genetics participates in population health in a proportion of 10–15%. The share of environment is about 20% and lifestyle participates in forming health or disease 50%. In the context of time and space, the phenomenon of nutrition and physical activities as a part of an environmental and lifestyle play a crucial role [31].

Recent research has focused on an enlarged set of factors in the development of lifestyle diseases. These factors include:

- Demographic factors (age, sex, and ethnic)
- Social and cultural factors (education, income)

- Biological factors (genetic, motherhood)
- Behavioral factors (physical activity, eating habits, smoking, and alcohol).

Lifestyle, and consequently also the structure of needs are the result of conditioning and choices of man, although for children, it is more often a question of conditioning rather choices. With age, the conditioning loses ground in favor of conscious choices. However, in childhood family and school are more important institutions that shape children's lifestyle.

Researchers ought to collaborate with schools to develop and implement interventions, and also to evaluate their impact on health and educational outcomes. In addition, the assessment and evaluation of interventions that promote physical activity and nutrition during school age are to be performed. Finally, these evaluations are to be more than simple measures of acceptability/fidelity and they include detailed contextual information to explicitly indicate what works, for whom, in what contexts and why [32].

In other words, obesity is an important worldwide health matter. Health precedence is to change eating and movement habits (to increase physical activity, restrict sedentary behavior and enhance the quality of nutrition). A little stress on health oriented education and lack of institutional support are barriers to healthier lifestyles of current population. Stronger cooperation between institutions that are responsible for health and education contributes essential to intervention success. If we would like to live long, happy, without difficulties and self-sufficiently, we have to change our lifestyle. It is necessary to check energy intake and energy output, avoid the stress, relax active, think positive and build self-respect, self-control and also self-satisfaction.

4. Previous empirical results

The aim of this chapter is to present some previous results obtained in empirical research conducted by the author. Three empirical works with different samples and tasks were selected. The first research shows the actual situation in health-oriented knowledge in graduates of elementary school education (15 years old children) and effectiveness of teaching health education as full-bodied school subject in contrast to previous form of teaching some health-oriented topics in more other subjects. These results should support the new form of gaining necessary knowledge related to desirable lifestyle. The second research deals with existing lifestyles in university students, there represent the best educated groups of the population. Therefore, we can take them as representatives of our society, there will have opportunity to form attitudes and habits of future generations. We can see strong and weak points in lifestyles of young adults (graduates of our educational system). The last research results document contribution of active lifestyle for some health, mental and physical aspects of life in adult population. We have to know benefits of physical activity for the life and these inventions should endorse education for health, not only in schools. The founded results are very important for a positive change in the health behavior—changes in physical activity, nutrition and health-oriented habits.

4.1 Health education in school

There are many objectives in children's schooling, among them include development of intellect, economic purposes of job preparation and social purposes such as social standards and morality as well and health education. In terms of health education, schools serve as a platform for students to learn and access necessary knowledge, skills, and attitudes for them to develop healthy interests and practices related to health as they navigate through the decision making in their teenage years.

Health education is currently taught as an independent subject with at least 2 lessons per week within the school educational programme by 76% of schools. 53% of schools use lessons with teacher and lectures with experts (policemen for addiction theme, firemen for topics about behavior in danger) for health education. Health education was presently implemented by most of the surveyed primary schools (as an independent school subject in at least three grades in the primary school = 6–9th grade) [33].

We made a set of didactic manuals on the topic of body care, self-concept, physical self-concept and physical activity in our research study and promoted by them lessons of health education in experimental classes [34]. We applied this didactic material in the seventh classes in regularly subject Health Education (2 h per week) in duration half-year and we check out their effectiveness. The final questionnaire survey verified knowledge and the comparison with the knowledge of pupils from the ninth classes came after (old teaching model - pupils got health oriented information in other subjects as biology, family education...).

The main objective of this research at primary school was the elaboration and subsequent verification of the effectiveness of didactic manuals for the subject health education (analysis of their contribution to improving the knowledge and skills of pupils. The research project searched for the answer to the question: Can the quality of pupil's knowledge be increased in connection with the teaching form (regular lessons with the help of new didactic manuals)?

The experimental group was constituted by seventh-grade pupils (average age of 12.5 years) of the Second primary school in Plzen (n = 53 children). All of them completed the input and output questionnaire survey. Personal interviews were successively conducted with selected pupils. The closing questionnaire was also completed in control group in ninth grade in age 14.7 years (n = 34 pupils) and, lastly, the knowledge was compared.

We used as the main method for evaluation of health-oriented knowledge the questionnaire with 17 questions, 12 of them were formulated as closed (answers on a 5-point scale), other five questions were open (pupils expressed their opinion and attitude). We collected the data twice - first, before the start of teaching, the second time, 6 months later. The second used questionnaire was composed of seven open questions.

Our research according to eating habits of boys and girls shows a lot of limits. The boys are eating and drinking more often sweets, smoked products, and sweet drinks. The eating habits of girls are different they drink more water and eat more vegetable and fruit than boys. Interestingly, 18% of boys and 8% of girls do not eat meat.

Also in physical activity of our samples, we founded reserves. Recommended 7 h per week (together with two lessons of physical education) completing 53% of children. Very low physical activity demonstrated 22% of children (20% with 1–2 h and 2% with 1 and less hours of individual physical activity).

The knowledge in all monitored aspects of health was significantly better in the experimental classes (with health education as a separate school subject) in contrast to control classes (with information about health-oriented knowledge in other subjects according to previous teaching model).

In summary the research confirmed the effectiveness of regular lessons of Health education - pupils' knowledge significantly improved during this form of education (the most the area of self-concept and benefits of physical activities). The knowledge of the seventh-grade pupils was significantly better in all aspects than those of the ninth-grade pupils. It is more effective to teach health-oriented themes in the separate school subject, not as less important part in other school subjects. It is better to teach and practice skills through physical tasks and practical goals. Memory is enhanced when a skill is performed physically and visually and when they attach emotions (such as competition and stress of deadlines) to a task, in comparison to simply writing notes down in front of a blackboard.

4.2 University students' lifestyles

The purpose of this empirical investigation [35] was to determine the relationship between selected personality characteristics and health-supporting behavior in university students in the Czech Republic. In addition, an analysis of decision making in their lifestyles was conducted. The underlying assumptions of developmental stages of adolescence and the dynamics of young adults were based upon the importance of a hierarchical value system and the relations to responsible behavior, focusing individual and societal influences. The requirement of the important part of health and its values in that phase of development can open the opportunity for a desirable behavior in the same way as for a disciplined individual lifestyle in the future. If basic principles of quality of life are not valued early, it will be very difficult to live a healthy lifestyle.

The sample included students at three major universities in the Czech Republic: Charles University, Prague; Masaryk University, Brno; and Palacky University, Olomouc. Students constitute one of the best-educated groups in every society. We can, therefore, consider them as representatives of our country, taking part in the formation of attitudes and habits of future generations. Students (N = 4292), aged between 18 and 29 years, answered a questionnaire.

The research project was conducted using the following measuring instruments: Questionnaire "Health, Sport and Body Concepts in Middle- and Eastern-Europe" [36] and "Scale of schematic body silhouettes" (Modification of Fallon and Rozin, 1985), "NEO Personality-questionnaire" with five factors [37] about basic personality factors: openness to experience, dutifulness, extroversion, kindness, and neuroticism, "Questionnaire to Life-satisfaction" [38].

Questionnaire, "Health, Sport and Body-concepts in Middle- and East- Europe" with 40 items for body- and health-supporting behavior - main-component analysis with oblique rotation Promax (value Kappa = 4). Results revealed 11 factors explaining 65% of the common variance: physical activity, personal hygiene and care of appearance, weight- and figure- control, optimal habits of healthy lifestyle, enjoyment of smoking, alcohol, drug and/or drug use, taking medicine, satisfaction with own body, attention to health issues, including prevention, alternative treatments, regular physician visits, and avoiding of body-contact and presentation of own nakedness.

Through a cluster analysis (method K-Means), the types of lifestyles were determined under use of the 11 factors, presented above, of health- and body-related behaviors. We identified six different types of lifestyles and qualified them based on their usefulness to improve health.

(1) Hypochondriac (22.5%)

These people paid immoderate attention for their bodies (appearance care, hygiene, and medicine). They assumed the responsibility for prevention and possible health challenges, often visited physicians, did not smoke and drink alcohol. Women were clearly more focused than men (9.3% men, 90.7% women) in this group. Exponents of this lifestyle were relatively often discovered in all faculties—the most we found were medical students, with many students also in social sciences. The outstanding hypochondriacs were represented as sport science-related majors.

(2) Conscientious people (20.3%)

Many factors were evidenced in this group—physical activities were part of their lives, they focused on their lifestyle, and sought preventative measures to improve. They were interested in their health and, while critiquing their bodies, accepted them. In this group, women were at a ratio of 1:2 (32.9% men, 67.1% women). These students were very careful, living healthy and aware according to relation to their health. Many of these health-conscious students were medical majors. In comparison, social science majors were less health-conscious than medical students.

(3) Barrelhouse loafers (17.6%)

Students in this group were worried about hygiene and physical appearance, were more physically passive, less concerned with their health, consumed alcohol overly and used drugs socially. The lifestyles and health were not important for this group (24.7% men, 75.3% women). Many representatives of this attitudes and behaviors were from social sciences, a relatively large number was also law and economics majors.

This lifestyle was represented less in sport science students.

(4) Good Examples (16.8%)

This group was higher than average in all items—students exercised regularly, paid attention to their weight and their physique were concerned with good nutrition and placed special emphasis on prevention. This group was mostly women (82.2% women, 17.8% men). The representatives of this style were comprised of many sport science and medical students. In contrast, representatives of this lifestyle very rarely included mathematical-technical and natural sciences majors.

(5) Sportsmen/pleasure lovers (12.5%)

These students spent many hours per week physically active, dedicating less attention to their lifestyles as well as on care of health and appearance, paying less attention to weight and physique, visiting physicians regularly but viewing their bodies critically. This group involved 59.7% males and 40.3% females. Most of the students in this category represented sport science majors, but not many included competitive athletes; a relative large number of these students were mathematical-technical majors. Noticeably absent were representatives from medical majors.

(6) Careless people (10.4%)

These people ignored themselves and their health, they were physically passive and had ambivalent or negative relationship to their own bodies; hygiene and appearance care were for them not important. This group was overwhelmingly male, with a ratio of 2:1 (63.4% men, 36.6 women). Most of those in this category were found to be mathematical-technical majors, whereas sport science majors were barely found.

As conclusion to University students lifestyles is possible to say that only two of the six explored lifestyles could be termed as "healthy" ("Good examples" and "Conscious people") in University student lifestyles in the Czech Republic. Students representing these lifestyles were largely engaged in positive behaviors, including those declared as health-supporting (physical activity, quality of life, limited consumption of addictive drugs, control of health challenges in daily life, attentiveness about health issues, and regular physician and health care professional consultation). Contrary to these healthy lifestyles are those who are labeled "barrelhouse loafers" and "careless people." Some criteria of health-supporting behaviors are described by the last types as "sportsmen/pleasure lovers" and "hypochondriacs." Students characterized by those types concerned themselves in only one of the investigated categories: "Sportsmen/Pleasure lover" involved physical activity; "Hypochondriacs" included lack of minimization of health risks. Other health-supporting habits were ignored by students. Results indicated these modes of living are not very effective in terms of health support. Approximately 40% of our sample successfully participated in healthy lifestyles, whereas 60% still have attention and care deficits relative to their own health.

4.3 Adult lifestyle and self-assessed body image

We observed and analyzed the relation to the body not as independent aspects of individual lifestyles but as the components of the basic body concept. Personal physical satisfaction can be the result of individual experiences linked to one's own body. In many situations, the social environment also becomes a factor. When perusing published information about participation in sports activities and its influence on one's own health, little is still known about the area of intentional, planned behaviors, which contribute to one's personal satisfaction. Perceptions about one's body are very important for positive change in health behaviors—changes in physical activity, nutrition, and health habits.

The main task of the research, "Physical self and health" [39], was to analyze benefits of physical activities for physical and mental feelings of well-being. We made a website for objective of this study, containing the questionnaire, "Self-concept, Quality of Life" (SQL), which concluded eight parts.

The subdivision, "My body and health," concentrated on: visual aspects, physical activity and fitness, hygiene and body care, nourishment and food consumed, physical health and sexual behaviors. This subdivision focused the body image, which was judged from several views: its importance for me, my contentment with it, my feeling of having it under control, possibility for change.

The subdivision, "My thoughts and feelings," concentrated on psychological aspects that took into consideration impressions, abilities to learn and to self-assess. It focused on self-confidence, opinion in relation to several matters, power to check and deal with troubles and stress. The questions locked on accepting the way I am, a life free from redundant anxiety, worry and tension, self-esteem, mental health, spirit, and independence of ideas and behavior. Personal meaning of these matters is evaluated as well as self-satisfaction, feeling of control and possibilities for change.

Cronbach's α (internal consistency) for our sample—male and female—ranged between 0.68 and 0.92, respectively. Content validity of the questionnaire was verified. The data were analyzed using NCSS program. We present in results the comparison between adult men and women and among active and passive groups (different levels of physical activity per week).

We analyzed physical self at 864 adults in age 18–60 years [39]. The analysis of physical and mental self-image according to sex and level of physical activities (active people have four and more hours of physical activities in a week) shows interesting differences. While physically more active females focused their attention on body care and hygiene, physical health and activity, less sporting females focused on hygiene, physical health and visual aspects of their bodies. The crucial aspects of physically active males related physical health, sports behavior and fitness, and also hygiene. Physically passive males focused on hygiene, physical health, and sexual life. The whole sample expressed the highest satisfaction with hygiene and body care. Higher rate of dissatisfaction was watched in the physically passive groups. Active people in our sample were mostly oriented on nutrition and eating habits. In general, males supposed physical aspects less important than females, and physically passive males were even less happy than women. Both active groups were more contented than passive groups. Physically active males represented the happiest group of all.

Sport active females and males perceived more to control their health status and body. Females noticed a significantly higher control over their behavior for fun and significantly more liveliness for alteration than males. This marked greater openness and consciousness of personal chances. All groups perceived the highest chances for fun via sport and physical activity participation. Sport participants believed they had greater opportunities of reaching all aspects, but males saw less opportunities than females. By mentioning few chances, passive groups also manifested specific skepticism in regard to personal possibility to change.

We also took interest in discovery differences in the perceptions and evaluation of health status, health matters, and health-related body care. The most frequently mentioned health trouble was backache, which was reported by nearly half of all female participants and as many as 80% of male partakers. Exhaustion, digestive complaints, and sleep disorders were quite often as well. In general, males had more health troubles than females (except headaches). Sport active groups reported significantly less complaints than the passive groups. The largest incongruity was found in exhausting and, in men, in digestive complaints. The positive results accomplished by the active respondents were conclusive.

In brief and in conclusion the results denote that physical self-concept is in large measure ascertained by the sex of the person rather than by other conditions. The self-concept and the feelings about myself (mental, physical, and also social) ride primarily on taking part in physical activity and less on age, education, and other factors. The sporting people were aware of body fitness and attractiveness and health status more, were also significantly satisfied with most aspects evaluated on physical and mental states. Simultaneously they felt more in check-up of their bodies and emotions. Active women saw more chances for change, which marked a higher level of self-confidence. Furthermore, the number of health troubles manifested by active part of sample was significantly lower than those mentioned by inactive adults.

5. Conclusion

This chapter demonstrated that there is a need to advocate for increases in physical activity and decreases in sedentary behavior. It is believed that a multi-level, multi-sectorial approach is required for this to be successful. This contribution brings some comparative findings in the European context and enriches the previous literature about lifestyle and education possibilities for improving health status and desirable behavior in contemporary population.

Society is now under media pressure, which demands that everybody take good care of their bodies without respecting individual possibilities and limits faced by every individual. Our task is to educate people to take qualified measures to improve their health and accept themselves the way they are. Success and socio-economic prosperity can be achieved only by a healthy society. A healthy society is composed of healthy individuals who recognize their own value, who accept themselves and who work on their own growth and development with their own individual limits. Regular physical activity brings numerous health benefits, such as reduced risks of cardiovascular disease, some types of cancer (e.g., breast and colon) and diabetes. It also helps to maintain the optimum body weight, improves the blood lipid profile, the digestive tract function and mental health (reduces stress, increases self-esteem and self-control and ability to concentrate) and boosts the body's immune system. Physical activity also helps to control already existing health problems (e.g., diabetes, high blood pressure or high cholesterol levels), and it is important for maintaining physical, mental and cognitive health in older age people. There is a link between physical activity and life expectancy physically active people tend to live longer than inactive ones. On the other hand, insufficient physical activity, along with poor eating habits, leads to an increase in obesity in the population and unhealthy life.

The best way to live healthier is to have reasons to move (instead of using escalators to go upstairs, instead to buy sweet cookies and drinks in school vending machine to bring fruit and vegetable from home, instead of going by the car as transport to the school and leisure activities to use bike or to walk, instead to sitting in front of the TV or computer for hours to move outsides for 1 h).

Another foundation for the improvement of lifestyles relies on some more conscious behavior supported from the government (less opportunities and more difficulties buying alcohol drinks, tobacco and other drugs, by breathing fresh air, by eating and drinking valuable and low-cost food and drinks, by using a variable type of movement and inexpensive leisure activities and also by providing education for healthy life in all generations).

Young generation is highly perceptive to the adoption of values, attitudes, and behaviors, which are offered by social environment. Therefore, it is very important in which social surroundings young people grow up. It is evident that the basis for possible changes to the health lifestyle is the revision of basic life values for a young generation.

Acknowledgements

We would like to thank all participants of the original studies that contributed data to this chapter (pupils at basic school in Plzen, university students from Prague, Olomouc and Brno, adults participated in questioning of "Self-concept and, quality of Life."

The realization of the study was supported by the scientific branch development program FTVS UK "Social sciences aspects of human movement studies" at the Charles University Prague as the part of project PROGRES n. Q19.

Author details

Ludmila Fialova
Charles University, Prague, Czech Republic

*Address all correspondence to: lidafialova@seznam.cz

References

[1] Bouchard C, Shephard RJ. Physical Activity, Fitness and Health. International Proceedings and Consensus Statement. Champaign: Human Kinetics; 1994

[2] World Health Organisation. Obesity and Overweight. 2014. Available from: http://www.who.int/mediacentre/factsheets/fs311/en/. [Accessed: 2017-01-12]

[3] U.S. Department of Health and Human Services: Physical Activity and Health: A Report of the Surgeon General. Atlanta, Georgia: U.S. Department of Health and Human Services, Centers for Disease Control and Prevention, National Center for Chronic Disease Prevention and Health Promotion; 1996

[4] Colley RC, Garriguet D, Janssen I, Craig C, Clarke J, Tremblay MS. Physical activity of Canadian children and youth: Accelerometer results from the 2007-2009 Canadian health measures survey. Health Reports. 2011;**22**:22. Statistics Canada, Catalogue no. 82-003-XPE

[5] Active Healthy Kids Canada. Active Kids Are Fit to Learn - Report Card on Physical Activity for Children and Youth. Toronto: Active Healthy Kids Canada; 2009

[6] Katzmarzyk PT, Church TS, Craig CL, Bouchard C. Sitting time and mortality from all causes, cardiovascular disease, and cancer. Medicine and Science in Sports and Exercise. 2009;**41**:998-1005

[7] Rychtecky A. Physical, sports, and health education against the sedentary lifestyles and obesity in Czech young people. In: Kai Chin M, editor. Physical Education and Health. Global Perspectives and Best Practice. USA: Sagamore Publishing; 2014. pp. 147-161

[8] Janssen I, Leblanc AG: Systematic review of the health benefits of physical activity and fitness in school-aged children and youth. International Journal of Behavioral Nutrition and Physical Activity. 2010;**7**:40

[9] Paterson D, Warburton D. Physical activity and functional limitations in older adults: A systematic review related to Canada's physical activity guidelines. International Journal of Behavioral Nutrition and Physical Activity. 2010;**7**:38

[10] Carpensen CJ, Powell KE, Christenson GM. Physical activity, exercise, and physical fitness: Definitions and distinctions for health-related research. Public Health Reports. 1985;**100**:126-131

[11] Marcus BH, Forsyth HL. Psychologie aktivního způsobu života: motivace lidí k pohybovým aktivitám. Praha: Portál; 2010

[12] Owen N, Bauman A, Brown W. Too much sitting: A novel and important predictor of chronic disease risk? British Journal of Sports Medicine. 2009;**43**(2):81-83

[13] Tremblay MS, Colley R, Saunders TJ, Healy GN, Owen N. Physiological and health implications of a sedentary lifestyle. Applied Physiology, Nutrition, and Metabolism. 2010;**35**:725-740

[14] American Academy of Pediatrics. Active healthy living: Prevention of childhood obesity through increased physical activity. Pediatrics. 2006;**117**(5):1834-1842

[15] Whitt-Glover MC, Taylor WC, Floyd MF, Yore MM, Yancey AK, Matthews CE. Disparities in physical activity and sedentary behaviours among US children and adolescents: Prevalence, correlates, and intervention

implications. Journal of Public Health Policy. 2009;**30**(Suppl 1):309-340

[16] Kenny E, Taoiseach A. Get Active! Physical Education, Physical Activity and Sport for Children and Young People: A Guiding Framework. Ireland: Department of Education and Skills; 2012

[17] Kirk SFL, PENNEY TL, LANGILLE JJ. The Relationship between Screen Time, Physical Activity, Dietary Intake and Healthy Weights in Children and Youth: Literature Review and Recommendations for Intervention. Halifax: Halifax Regional Physical Activity and the IWK Health Centre. Nova Scotia Department of Health Promotion and Protection; 2009

[18] Whitlock EP, O'Connor EA, Williams SB, Beil TL, Lutz KW. Effectiveness of weight management interventions in children: A targeted systematic review for the USPSTF. Pediatrics. 2010;**125**:396-418

[19] Healthy People. Understanding and Improving Heath. Washington, DC: U.S. Government Printing Office; 2010

[20] Physical Activity Guidelines Advisory Committee. Physical Activity Guidelines Advisory Committee Report. Washington, DC: U.S. Department of Health and Human Services; 2008

[21] Slepička P, Mudrák J, Slepičková I. Sport a pohyb v životě seniorů. Praha: Karolinum; 2015

[22] Eurobarometr. 2014. Available from: http://ec.europa.eu/commfrontoffice/publicopinion//indexb_en.htm [Accessed: 2018-11-23]

[23] Raport about the Health of Czech citizens. 2014. Available from: http://www.mzcr.cz/verejne/dokumenty/zprava-o-zdravi-obyvatel-ceske-republiky2014-_9420_3016_5.html. [Accessed: 2017-01-14]

[24] World Health Organization. Office for Europe. Obesity. 2012. Available from: http://www.euro.who.int/en/what-we-do/health-opics/noncommunicablediseases/obesity. [Accessed: 2017-01-12]

[25] Diener E. Mint: Subjective well-being. Psychological Bulletin. 1984;**95**:542-575

[26] Kasser T. Materialism and its Alternatives (I.S. Csikszentmihalyi). A Life Worth Living: Contributions to Positive Psychology. Oxford: University Press; 2006

[27] Kelder SH, Perry CL, Klepp KI. Mint: Community- wide youth exercise promotion: Long- term outcomes of the Minnesota heart health program and the class of 1989 study. The Journal of School Health. 1993;**63**:218-223

[28] Jeřábek J, Tupý J. Framework Educational Programme (Rámcový vzdělávací program). Praha: VUP; 2007

[29] Fialova L. Differences in body image and health among sport active and passive adults as a base for school health education. American Journal of Educational Research. 2014;**2**:782-787

[30] Eurostat. 2016. Available from: http://ec.europa.eu/eurostat/data/statistics-a-z/abc [Accessed: 2018-1-26]

[31] Health 2020 – National Strategy for Health Protection and Promotion and Disease Prevention. Praha: Ministry of Health of the Czech Republic; 2014

[32] Langford R, Bonell CH, Jones H, Campbell R. Obesity prevention and the health promoting schools framework: Essential components and barriers to success. International Journal of Behavioral Nutrition and Physical Activity. 2015;**129**:167-171

[33] Fialová L, Flemr L, Marádová E, Mužík V. Vzdělávací oblast Člověk

a zdraví v současné škole. Praha: Karolinum; 2014

[34] Hájková L. Health education in the primary school/ Výchova ke zdraví na základní škole. Diploma thesis. Praha: UK FTVS; 2012

[35] Dosedlová J, Fialová L, Kebza V, Slováčková Z. Prerequisites of Health and Life Satisfaction/ Předpoklady zdraví a životní Spokojenosti. Brno: MSD; 2008

[36] Mrazek J, Fialová L, Bychovskaja I. Sport, health and body concepts in central and eastern Europe. Journal of Comparative Physical Education and Sport. 1982;**2**:52-56

[37] Costa PT, Mc Crae RR. Influence of extraversion and neuroticism on subjective well- being: Happy and unhappy people. Journal of Personality and Social Psychology. 1980;**38**:668-678

[38] Pavot W, Diener E. Review of the satisfaction with life scale. Psychological Assessment. 1993;**5**:164-172

[39] Fialová L. Personal satisfaction, physical self and health related behaviour from the aspect of involvement in sports in adult population. In: Louková T, Hátlová B, Adámková M, editors. Psychomotor Therapy. Ústí Nad Labem: University of J. E. Purkyně; 2015. pp. 55-66

Chapter 6

The Role of Exercise in Reducing PTSD and Negative Emotional States

Robert Motta

Abstract

There is considerable research indicating that exercise can be of significant benefit in reducing anxiety and depression. There are far fewer investigations of the role of exercise in reducing posttraumatic stress disorder (PTSD). This chapter reviews empirical research on the impact of exercise, particularly aerobic exercise, in reducing PTSD and negative emotional states. A variety of models are reviewed to possibly explain why exercise is so beneficial. Those who suffer from PTSD are notoriously treatment avoidant. Exercise is presented as an effective intervention for PTSD, anxiety, and depression and because it does not produce the level of avoidance that traditional psychotherapies do, it becomes a valuable potential tool for treating PTSD.

Keywords: posttraumatic stress disorder, anxiety, depression, exercise

1. Introduction: the effect of exercise on posttraumatic stress disorder (PTSD)

In the early days of research on the impact of exercise on negative emotional states, there was fairly consistent evidence of its beneficial impact [1, 2]; but there was virtually no evidence of its utility in managing PTSD. The reasoning behind the lack of evidence for the utility of exercise in reducing PTSD was that PTSD is a far more complex and enduring problem than many of the more transitory disorders such as anxiety and depression. PTSD literally transforms the individual sufferer on virtually all levels. It is not as simple as fear of driving on highways but involves an alteration of one's sense of self and one's view of the environment. PTSD sufferers report that they are no longer the person they once were and they no longer see the world in the same way. It seemed that exercise could not have a real impact on such a pervasive and enduring disorder as PTSD. I was somewhat taken by surprise when one of my doctoral students was able to prove otherwise [3].

In her study Dr. Manger obtained a sample of individuals from the community who had experienced a variety of traumatic events including the tragic death of a loved one or friend, a sexual or physical assault, serious accident (most common were automobile accidents), combat, severe illness or disease, or injury. Study participants reported experiencing between two and six traumatic events and on average were 48 years of age. Participants were then required to walk or jog on a treadmill at a moderate intensity level for 30 minutes and then engage in a cool down for 10 minutes. Moderate intensity exercise was defined as 60–80% of maximum heart rate for half an hour. Heart rate monitors were provided. Participants agreed to exercise two to three times per week for 10 weeks. Overall results showed significant reductions in PTSD, anxiety and depression following the exercise intervention. These results were maintained during the one-month follow-up period. In the exercise intervention presented here there was no need for those involved to deal with traumatic experiences other than, that which may have been encountered in filling out paper and pencil measures of trauma, and answering questions during initial interview. The reductions in negative emotional states that followed the exercise intervention cannot be attributed to any traditional form of therapeutic intervention as none was offered in this study. It appeared that exercise alone was responsible for the reductions in PTSD, anxiety and depression. This of course begs the question, which may be unanswerable: why does exercise have a beneficial effects noted here. To date there seems to be no universally agreed upon answer.

1.1 Additional empirical studies of exercise and PTSD

Another more recent study of adults, focusing specifically on women veterans of childbearing age, was conducted to determine if exercise in and of itself could positively impact PTSD [4]. The protocol involved brisk walking at a rate of 3 miles/hour for 30–40 minutes, 4 days a week for a total of 12 weeks. The exercise duration was gradually increased upward in the first 3 weeks to a full duration of 30–40 minutes per session by the end of week 3. Exercise sessions had a 3–5 minute warm up before advance the walking speed to its targeted intensity level. Results again showed significant reductions in PTSD and depression, and increases in quality of life measures and pain reduction. The authors state: "Finally, for patients with prominent avoidance related to their traumatic events, exercise many provide a safe and structured activity than can address social isolation and promote recovery" (p. 1813).

Avoidance is a major problem in treating PTSD with traditional treatments that require the patient to re-confront and reprocess their trauma experiences. If interventions, such as exercise can be effective in reducing this disorder and do not place a heavy emphasis on re-confronting prior trauma, they have an important place in our treatment choices. No study is without its limitations including this one which did not have a comparison group that was diagnosed PTSD but was not receiving exercise. Nevertheless, the overall thrust of existing empirical investigations certainly seems to point toward exercise as an effective intervention for PTSD.

The majority of research studies on exercise and PTSD, including those presented to this point use a cross-sectional approach whereby a group of individuals, most often adults, with PTSD are enrolled in an exercise program for a specific period and are given pre and posttest measures to see if there have been reductions in negative emotional states. In contrast an online longitudinal study involving 182 individuals who screened positive for PTSD [5] was conducted. In addition to a measure of PTSD participants completed online assessments of exercise behavior, psychological distress, sleep quality, pain, and alcohol/substance abuse. Findings were that there was a significant and direct effect of exercise on avoidance/numbing symptoms of PTSD. This is of no small significance as avoidance is one of the major difficulties in treating those who are traumatized. Numbing refers to emotional dampening and lack of engagement. However, for those who engaged in strenuous intensity exercise, which was defined as vigorous running or cycling, there was significantly less avoidance/numbing and hyperarousal. Those who engaged in strenuous exercise activity also reported better sleep quality, reduced substance abuse, less pain, and a reduction in overall PTSD symptoms than those who were less active.

Overall results of this study point to beneficial effects of aerobic activity particularly for those who exercise vigorously. However, this should not be interpreted to mean that moderate levels of exercise are not of value. The general message from the research literature is that even moderate levels of exercise are effective in reducing both anxiety and depression. Given that anxiety and depression are key components of PTSD, it should be clear that encouraging patients to exercise is generally excellent practice.

There are those who claim that the beneficial effects of exercise may be due to changes in brain morphology, chemistry, and function. These beneficial effects include improved learning and memory, anti-depressant and anti-anxiety effects, reduced cognitive decline related to aging, and improvements in symptoms of neurodegenerative diseases. Exercise appears to improve mood and cognition and to have its greatest effects on the hippocampus where both neurogenesis (nerve cell growth), angiogenesis (increase blood availability through the growth of new blood vessels) have been shown. Although the exact molecular mechanisms responsible for the exercise-induced neuroplasticity needs to be further researched, progress is continuing in this area especially regarding studies of neurotransmitter systems.

Another study [6] examined active and inactive adolescent and adult twins between the ages of 14–24 with diagnosable anxiety disorders. Results showed that exercise reduced anxiety, PTSD, agoraphobia, and other specific phobias in the physically active twin. Twins not engaging in exercise did not have reductions in these disorders. The value of this study is that it helps to nullify genetic explanations as to why individuals may benefit from exercise. The authors kept the genetic factor relatively constant and continued to find that exercise alone benefited the active twin.

1.2 Exercise and PTSD in adolescents

Having found positive results for the impact of aerobic exercise on PTSD in adults, the next step was to determine if the same outcome would occur in an adolescent sample. We recruited participants from a residential treatment center who were female, who had primarily been physically abused, sexually abused, maltreated or some combination of those, were between the ages of 14–17, and who had a diagnosis of PTSD based upon standardized measures [7]. Participants engaged in a structured group aerobic exercise program for 40 minutes, three times per week for a total of 8 weeks. The form of exercise varied with some girls jogging and some doing kickboxing but all of which produced an aerobic effect. Measures of PTSD, anxiety, and depression were taken twice during the beginning and end of a baseline period in which no intervention took place, at the end of the exercise intervention, and at a one-month follow up. Once again, results provided support for the positive effects of aerobic exercise on reducing PTSD, anxiety, and depression. Fewer youngsters met the criteria for PTSD and the end of the study than at the beginning and overall, significant reduction in anxiety and depression were shown. One of the major values of the exercise intervention is that it achieved positive therapeutic outcomes without the need for the adolescents to engage in formal therapy, which they were reluctant to do. It is easy to see that adolescent females may have been immensely troubled by their abuse and avoidant as far as sharing information in a formal therapeutic setting. If significant symptom reduction can be attained by a simple aerobic exercise activity, such activity should become part of the formal structure of interventions for these youngsters.

Finding that PTSD could be reduced through simple aerobic exercise interventions within adult and adolescent samples, another study [8] was conducted with youngsters 14–17 years of age at a private residential treatment facility, but this time the attempt was made to use only moderate intensity walking as the form of intervention rather than using varied forms of more intense aerobic activity. In this study, participants completed a 5 week baseline and then an intervention which involved 25 minutes sessions of exercise which included: 1 minute of slow leisurely walking (warm up), 23 minutes of moderated intensity walking, and 1 minute of slow leisurely walking (cool down). Heart rates were maintained at 60–90% of maximum. By keeping the intervention unvaried and structured, the hope was to make the study more precise than earlier conducted investigations. The majority of participants showed statistically significant reductions in PTSD symptoms from baseline to post-intervention. There was also a reduction in trauma related stress. Results of anxiety and depression measures were not as clear cut as those from PTSD and this may have been due to the fact that initial levels were not overly high and therefore significant reductions were less likely to occur. Like previous studies, the reductions in PTSD were primarily maintained in follow-up and in some cases the reductions increased over time.

The authors concluded that aerobic exercise interventions might be appropriate for youngsters who demonstrate difficulty with expressing their emotions verbally as is required in traditional CBT type therapies. In addition, aerobic exercise as an intervention for PTSD may be more appropriate than exposure therapies, which is more likely to be tolerated in teens with concentration problems, self-control difficulty, and with histories of sexual-abuse and the avoidance of discussing their traumatic experiences that such abuse usually produces.

A study of adolescent females [9] suggested that peer pressures related to social acceptance significantly affect the high level of anxiety in this group. Issues such as wearing fashionable clothes, having a boyfriend, doing well in school, being popular etc. were factors upon which their peers judged their merit. In this study, individuals in the exercise group participated in 50 minute dance classes, four times a week, for 4 weeks. The classes followed a dance routine to elevate heart rate to 160 beats per minute and ended with a cool-down to bring the heart rate down to 100 beats per minute. Results of the study showed clear benefits in terms of anxiety reduction by engaging in the aerobic dance routine. Thus it appears that a variety of exercises from treadmills, to walking, to kickboxing to dance and others can have beneficial effects on negative emotional states.

2. Why does exercise help with PTSD and emotional disorders?

The short answer to this question is that no one knows for sure why exercise is beneficial in reducing PTSD and the anxiety and depression that accompany this disorder. There are a number of hypotheses, none of which are universally accepted.

2.1 Thermogenic hypothesis

This hypothesis proposes that exercise creates an elevation in body temperature and this has a beneficial impact on emotional states. Specifically, aerobic forms of exercise are said to raise the temperature of brain regions such as the brain stem and this produces a tranquilizing effect along with muscle tension reduction. The hypothesis has specifically been used to explain anxiety reduction rather than depression and PTSD. However, given that PTSD was formerly classified as an anxiety disorder and anxiety is a major component of PTSD, it stands to reason that exercise would have a beneficial impact on PTSD. One of the difficulties with the thermogenic hypothesis is that temperature elevation might be an intervening variable that has little to do with the beneficial emotional impact of exercise. For example, it may be that exercise increases temperature but also alters neurochemistry and it is the latter that produces the benefit, not temperature elevation per se. From this perspective temperature plays a correlational rather than a causal role. Additionally, living in a warm environment has not been shown to reduce depression, anxiety, or PTSD nor does having a fever, which also increases internal body temperature. The thermogenic hypothesis does not appear to have held up well as an explanation for the beneficial effects on emotion resulting from exercise.

2.2 The endorphin and endocannabinoid hypotheses

Perhaps the most popular explanation for the positive impact on mood that results from exercise is the endorphin hypothesis. This hypothesis is based on the observation that following vigorous exercise of one half hour or more, there is an elevation of a special endogenous opiate (*B*, or beta, endorphin). This endogenous or body produced opiate is released through exercise and is said by some to be responsible for the "runners high," an elevation of mood following running or jogging or extended periods. The endorphin hypothesis is not without its critics who have carefully examined the data from empirical studies.

One such study compared a jogging group to a relaxation group that did not engage in exercise to a group that did back stretches. The moods that were examined were anger, tension, energy level, calmness, positive mood, depression and others. While all groups produced positive emotional changes there were no differences among the groups. If beta-endorphin is released through exercise, the non-exercise groups should not have shown positive changes and yet they did. Clearly something other than, or in addition to endorphins must be responsible for positive emotional effects of exercise.

A further critique of the endorphin hypothesis is that circulating endorphin levels are not reflective of brain endorphin levels and endorphins cannot cross the blood brain barrier. So even if circulating or peripheral endorphin levels increased, this should not have an impact on brain mediated emotional states. A further critique of the endorphin hypothesis is that when the endorphin blocking substance naloxone, an opiate antagonist, is provided to those experiencing the runners high, the elevation in mood is not diminished. If endorphins were causal to exercise induced mood changes, one would expect a significant deterioration in mood following naloxone injection.

It may be of some significance to note here that a recent alternative to the endorphin hypothesis has come to be known as the *endocannabinoid hypothesis*. Endocannabinoids are bodily produces substances that are similar in action to that of tetrahydrocannabinol (THC), the active constituent in marijuana. Using trained male college students running on a treadmill or cycling on a stationary bike for 50 minutes at 70–80% of maximum heart rate, elevations of endocannabinoids were detected in blood plasma. Because activation of the endocannabinoid system reduces pain sensations, it has been suggested that this might be what is behind the runners high and alterations of mental and emotional processes [10]. Owing to the presence of cannabinoid receptors in the skin, lung, and muscle, it has been suggested that there may be a role for endocannabinoids in producing analgesic effects through exercise. Unlike the endorphin hypothesis where it was noted that endorphins do not cross the blood brain barrier, cannabinoids do appear to operate both centrally (i.e., in the central nervous system) and in the peripheral nervous system. Cannabinoids are reported to reduce anxiety, alter attention, and impair working memory, much like THC does. So, although research is in the early phases, endocannabinoids have been proposed as an alternative to endorphins as the possible mediator of the runners high, analgesic effects and beneficial psychological effects of exercise. The endocannabinoid hypothesis is of comparatively recent development and is not anywhere near as widely accepted as the apparently doubtful endorphin hypothesis.

2.3 Monoamine hypothesis

This hypothesis is somewhat similar to the endorphin and endocannabinoid hypotheses in that is proposes that exercise produces chemical changes in the body and these are what causes mood changes in exercise. The monoamine hypothesis proposes that exercise results in increased brain availability of brain neurotransmitters such as serotonin, dopamine, and norepinephrine and that these result in reductions in depression and other negative emotional states. Available studies show that while exercise does result in monoamine elevations as assessed in plasma and urine, the question remains as to whether there similar elevations in the brain take place. In fact testing of biochemical hypotheses is difficult in humans because it often involves invasive procedures such as spinal taps for cerebrospinal fluid samples. Further, biochemical samples obtained from blood or other body fluids may not necessarily reflect the availability of similar biochemical samples in the brain. Animal studies suggest that exercise increases serotonin and norepinephrine in the brain but reliable and replicable studies in humans have not been demonstrated.

Another line of reasoning that further clouds the issue of whether biochemical changes following exercise is causal of positive mood enhancement is that all mental activity is in essence chemical activity of the nervous system, especially the central nervous system. So, as will soon be discussed, it may be possible that positive mood states arise from perceptions of having successfully completed some form of strenuous activity, and the positive mental state is what drives the biochemical changes, rather than the other way around. The issue is, what is responsible for causing what? Which came first?

2.4 Distraction hypothesis

This hypothesis suggests that psychological or environmental changes are what are responsible for changes in emotional states following exercise and that biochemical mediators play an ancillary role. The hypothesis proposes that when one is engaged in vigorous physical activity it is difficult to simultaneously entertain depressive thoughts and negatively tinged depressive ruminations. We only have so much attention to go around and when one is busy exercising there is little available attention for depressive rumination. It is usually when one is inactive, immobile, and has few demands on one's time that there is time and space available to engage in depressive thoughts. And, as we saw earlier, negative thinking and cognitive distortions are the basis for negative emotional states according to CBT perspectives.

In some studies exercise has been compared to control groups such as relaxation training, or waiting list controls, where one is distracted yet not involved in physical activity. The results of these studies are varied with some showing reductions in depression following distracting activity and some not. However, when one examines mood elevation and not simply reduction in depression, usually exercise shows greater changes than non-exercise interventions. So, it is possible that distraction serves as a means through which one moves away from depressive rumination, but that for mood elevation to occur, distraction may not be a sufficiently effective means.

2.5 Self-efficacy theory

Self-efficacy perceptions refer to one's self-view of their capabilities to accomplish certain objectives. The originator of self-efficacy theory [11], claims that people who are depressed are comparatively lacking in a healthy sense of self-efficacy. Those who are clinically depressed see themselves as relatively incapable of setting goals and accomplishing hoped for objectives. These negative self-perceptions eventuate in depressive rumination on, for example, perceived inadequacies, and these perceptions decrease the possibility of engaging in self-validating behaviors.

The studies that have been conducted do in fact show that when one engages in physical exercise they feel more accomplished and more capable of achieving various exercise related goals. Their self-efficacy perceptions, i.e., their view of themselves setting specific exercise targets and accomplishing them has been found to increase following a planned sequence of exercise. The research however, on whether these enhanced views of exercise competence can produce reductions in clinical depression is less clear-cut. It does seem clear that exercise is associated with reductions in depression and elevation in mood. Whether these outcomes are due to alterations in one's self-perceptions of their capabilities is less obvious.

2.6 Conclusion on causal hypotheses of exercise effects

At this point it is unclear as to whether biochemical or psychological factors mediate the positive effects of exercise on mood states such as depression. Depression and anxiety are significant factors in PTSD and the alleviation of the emotional distress that they cause would be a productive step in treating PTSD. It may very well be that we are making an error in seeking out unitary causes for the beneficial effects of exercise and that a combination of biochemistry, psychology, and perhaps even socialization, and in some instances, spiritual issues come into play, and maybe these vary in importance depending on at what point in one's cycle of emotional distress one chooses to intervene. What we can derive from the available literature is that exercise alleviates emotional distress.

Why this is so is, as of this writing, unclear. However, from a practical point of view, it does seem that exercise produces biochemical alterations in the nervous system, even if the specific nature of these biochemical events is unclear, and it is these biochemical changes that improve negative emotional states. Perhaps a biochemical and self-efficacy interpretation in combination is the most useful model of the beneficial effects of exercise.

2.7 From research to clinical perspectives

Those clinicians who have treated individuals suffering from PTSD, anxiety, and depression know that it is a real challenge to get them to engage in exercise, despite its beneficial effects. The American College of Sports Medicine recommends that those between the ages of 18–65 should engage in moderate intensity exercise for 30 minutes 5 days a week. Moderate exercise intensity is defined as 60–80% of maximum heart rate. In general maximum heart rate has been calculated as 220 minus age multiplied by .6 to .8 So, for an individual who is 50 the calculation would be $220 - 50 = 170$; $170(.6) = 102$; $170(.8) = 136$. Therefore the 50 year old should exercise in such a way that they maintain a heart rate of 102–136 for half an hour, 5 days a week. Is this reasonable?

The numbers presented above, exercising 5 days a week for a half hour at moderate intensity are, for all intents and purposes, unrealistic, to say the least, for many and especially for those who are depressed. Getting a depressed patient to do anything, other than that which is absolutely necessary to get on with their lives, is often a real challenge. So what is realistic? In many instances just getting them to go for a walk for 10 minutes or so maybe twice a week might be a major accomplishment. The idea is to start at a non-challenging level as most emotionally troubled patients are not physically fit, unmotivated, and resistant to physical activity. Start slow, be encouraging and move up the exercise level slowly. Baby steps are the guiding principle here. Start emotionally distressed patients with something they might see as enjoyable. A 10 minute stroll in the park might be a suitable starting point. Certainly, a moderate to vigorous intensity level three to five times per week is likely to have a psychologically beneficial effect, but if the exercise demands become overwhelming to a patient, which they easily can, not only will the patient become discouraged, but they may also begin to believe that their therapist does not understand them and is out of touch. The patient's inability to accomplish exercise goals may likely be seen as a failure and this failure further validates a negative, depressive self-view. As in treating PTSD, the mantra here is to move slowly, and at a pace the patient can tolerate.

2.8 Childhood negative affectivity and PTSD reduction through exercise

With the exception of the few studies noted above involving older children and early adolescents, there are few studies that examine the impact of exercise, anxiety, depression, and PTSD in children and yet anxiety and depression are key components of PTSD. It has been noted [12] that only about 36% of children and adolescents participate in physical education and this is unfortunate given the beneficial effects that exercise appears to have in relation to emotional disorders. The few exercise interventions that have been implemented with children do, in fact show that there is an exercise—anxiety reduction relationship. In a study involving children [13] 9–12 year olds engaged in physical activity, resistance training, and stretching for 12 weeks. Exercise resulted in reductions in anxiety, negative mood, and improvements in physical self-concept, and overall self-concept. There have been additional studies that correlated exercise among children with improvements in grades, standardized test scores, and feelings of well-being.

There are literally hundreds of empirical studies showing that exercise significantly reduces depression in adult samples and often to a degree equal to or greater than traditional cognitive therapies and psychotropic medication. As a result, there can be little doubt about the utility of exercise as an adjunct to traditional therapies or a stand-alone intervention for reducing depression. The problem with prescribing exercise, as clinicians are all too aware, is that the more depressed a person is the less likely they are to engage in exercise. They simply lack the energy or motivation to go to a gym or go outside and engage in brisk walking, jogging, or perhaps swimming. The research on childhood and adolescent depression is far less abundant than that of adults.

Children and adolescents who are depressed experience prolonged or temporary sadness, reduced interest in normal activity, negative and self-critical self-evaluation, difficulties in concentration and memory, socialization difficulties, and impairment in everyday functioning. In the United States, up to 2.5% or children and 8.3% of adolescents suffer from depression. The problems of depressed youngsters can extend well past childhood and lead to substance abuse and suicide. Approximately 7% of adolescents who develop major depressive disorder, later commit suicide as young adults. In addition to the treatment options of traditional psychotherapies and medication, physical activity has been researched as an alternative for these youngsters.

A correlational study [14] examined the relationships among self-reported exercise levels, depression, and a number of other interpersonal characteristics including relationship with parents and peers, sports involvement, drug use, and academic performance. A sample of high school seniors completed questionnaires and, on the basis of their answers, were divided into two groups: low exercise and high exercise. It was found that the high-exercise group reported significantly less depression, lower drug use and better relationships than the low-exercise group. While exercise appeared to produce these positive outcomes, it could be argued that those who were less depressed were more likely to have already been engaging in these positive behaviors, unlike the previously depressed individuals. The problems establishing causality from correlational studies are well known.

In contrast to the above correlational study, typical experimental studies randomly assign participants into groups: those who receive treatment and those who do not. Data are gathered before and after the intervention, and the participants' results are compared to one another. Doing so allows researchers to make inferences about the impact of the treatment, in this case exercise, on depressive symptomology. Another study [15] implemented an after school physical activity program with children 9–12 years of age. After assessing for depressed mood, the youngsters engaged in cardiovascular and resistance exercises three times per week for 12 weeks or did not engage in exercise. Upon completion of the study a significant reduction in depression was found for the exercise group.

A further investigation [16] examined the impact of a physical activity program on the psychological wellbeing of low-income Hispanic 4th grade children. A sample of children participated in a 6-week program. They were assigned to an aerobic group involving stationary bicycling, track running, and jumping on a trampoline or a control group that participated in shooting basketballs, walking, and playing foursquare. Pre and posttest depression scores were obtained and at the end of the intervention the aerobic group reported significantly less depression than the control group. The effect size of −.97 indicates a large impact of exercise on depression in this experimentally based study.

While the general thrust of the research shows that physical activity is associated with a significant reduction in depression, there are some who maintain that exercise can be a preventive measure as well. In contrast to other strategies that adolescents often use (substance use, emotional coping, and aggressive behavior), physical activity was found to decrease the likelihood of future depressive episodes. Again, this suggests that physical education programs within the schools can be a real benefit in promoting both physical and mental in youngsters.

3. Conclusion: implications of using exercise to impact anxiety, depression and PTSD

There is abundant and ever increasing evidence that exercise can be of significant benefit in reducing adult affective disorders including PTSD. There are literally hundreds of empirical studies demonstrating the beneficial effects of exercise on adult anxiety and depression and these are major components of PTSD. There are also a growing number of studies showing that exercise can beneficially impact adult PTSD directly. The emerging research shows that it can be of value for adolescents and children. The benefit of physical exercise in reducing negative affect is that exercise fits within the natural ecology if childhood and adolescent activity. In contrast psychotherapy and psychotropic medication are alien to youngsters. Physical education classes often exist within their schools so exercise is seen as an integral part of the educational process and part of what it means to be student within the school system.

Further work is needed to develop empirically sound methodologies for investigating the role of exercise in dealing with PTSD and other affective disorders. Exercise has long been seen as being of value for the physical wellbeing of children, adolescents, adults, and seniors. Empirical findings indicate that exercise has beneficial effects on psychological functioning as well. Further research should examine its benefits as a method of prevention for children and adolescents at risk for internalizing disorders, i.e., troubling emotional states that do not find outward expression.

Author details

Robert Motta
Hofstra University, Hempstead, New York, United States

*Address all correspondence to: motta9182@gmail.com

References

[1] Altchiler LS, Motta RW. Effects of aerobic and nonaerobic exercise on anxiety, absenteeism, and job satisfaction. Journal of Clinical Psychology. 1994;**50**:829-840

[2] Stein PN, Motta RW. Effects of aerobic and non aerobic exercise on depression and self-concept. Perceptual and Motor Skill. 1992;**74**:79-89

[3] Manger TA, Motta RW. The impact of an exercise program on posttraumatic stress disorder, anxiety, and depression. International Journal of Emergency Mental Health. 2005;**7**(1):49-57

[4] Shivakumar G, Anderson EH, Suris AM, North CS. Exercise for PTSD in women veterans: A proof of concept study. Military Medicing. 2017;**182**:1809-1814

[5] Whitworth JW, Craft LL, Dunsiger SI, Ciccolo JT. Direct and indirect effects of exercise on posttraumatic stress disorder symptoms: A longitudinal study. General Hospital Psychiatry. 2017;**49**:56-62

[6] De Moor MHM, Beem AL, Stubbe DI, Boomsma EJC, DeGeus EJ. Regular exercise, anxiety, depression, and personality: A population-based study. Preventive Medicine. 2006;**42**:273-279

[7] Newman CL, Motta RW. The effects of aerobic exercise on childhood PTSD, anxiety, and depression. International Journal of Emergency Mental Health. 2007;**36**:55-65

[8] Diaz AB, Motta RW. The effect of an aerobic exercise program on posttraumatic stress disorder symptom severity in adolescents. International Journal of Emergency Mental Health. 2008;**10**(1):49-60

[9] Silvestri L. Anxiety reduction though aerobic dance and progressive relaxation training. Education. 2001;**108**:34-40

[10] Dietrich A, McDaniel WF. Endocannabinoids and exercise. British Journal of Sports Medicine. 2004;**38**:536-541

[11] Bandura A. Self-Efficacy: The Exercise of Control. New York, NY: WH Freeman & Company; 1994

[12] Paluka SA, Schwenk TL. Physical activity and mental health current concepts. Sports Medicine. 2000;**29**:167-180

[13] Annesi J. Improvements in self-concept associated wit reductions in negative mood in preadolescents enrolled in an after school physical activity program. Psychological Reports. 2005;**97**:400-404

[14] Field T, Diego M, Sanders CE. Exercise Is Positively Related to Adolescents' Relationships and Academics. Scientific Research. 2001;**36**:105-110

[15] Anessi J. Relationship between self-efficacy and changes in rated tension and depression for 9-12 old children enrolled in a 12 week afterschool physical activity program. Perceptual and Motor Skills. 2004;**99**:191-194

[16] Crews DJ, Lochbaum MR, Landers DM. Aerobic physical activity effects on psychological well-being in low income Hispanic children. Perceptual and Motor Skills. 2004;**98**:319-324

Chapter 7

Social Inequalities, Poverty and Obesity

Vanessa Alves Ferreira and Rosana Magalhães

Abstract

Nowadays, the growth of obesity, especially in socially vulnerable groups, reveals the complex nature of food patterns involving socioeconomic and cultural aspects. In this scenario, there has been slow progress in intervention actions for this issue. In general, initiatives to reduce obesity tend to focus on changes in diet behavior and individual sector strategies. They underestimate broader aspects social inequalities, symbolic dynamics and cultural local situations. Faced with this reality, the objective of this study was to investigate the phenomenon of obesity in a context marked by poverty incorporating the constructivist perspective. About 24 interviews and 3 focus groups were performed. The expectation was to analyze perceptions, interpretations and practices around food and body fat. The results revealed fundamental components to be observed in the design of public policies aimed at the reduction of obesity. Concentrating in this direction, actions directed to the promotion of social equity and gender equality, as well as greater access to food, education, technology and the quality of health care, especially in the post-partum period, seems more promising ways of dealing with the problem of obesity in this local context.

Keywords: obesity, poverty, public policy

1. Introduction

In Brazil, the tendency of obesity in contexts marked by poverty and inequalities were studied [1–5]. Such analyzes may be valuable contributions to the deepening and understanding of the phenomenon of obesity in these segments, because they reveal the complex network of interrelationships that operate in this multifaceted dynamics of a more comprehensive and relational approach [5]. Explanations for obesity among the poor in Brazil are therefore interrelated with a number of important structural, economic, social and cultural transformations verified in the last that profoundly altered the relationship between Brazilians and food, body and health. In general terms, it can be said that these changes are linked to the emergence of obesogenic environments, that is, social, economic and cultural trends that stimulate the population to overeating and poor physical activity [5, 6].

Limitations of economic and social order also promoted inequalities in accessing the main means of intervention in the problem. Inequalities in access to healthy food and recreational public spaces have accentuated health inequalities, especially with in relation to the problem of obesity among the poor in Brazil. Thus, the limited choice of lifestyles that favor health and well-being promote marked inequalities in the daily life of these segments. Yet, income ratio does not seem to be the only factor or the most consistent to explain the phenomenon of obesity among the poor. Cultural conceptions related to food, body, health, work and living conditions permeate the dynamic [5, 6].

At the same time, the poor have been targeted by the market for unhealthy products, contributing to the growth profile of obesity. Companies that produce consumer goods, including processed and ultraprocessed foods, soft drinks and sugary drinks, among others, have been able to change behaviors and lifestyles, contributing to the increase of excess weight and its comorbidities in different groups, including those with lower income [7, 8]. This imposes protectionist measures of the Brazilian government aimed at regulating unhealthy products and expanding the supply of products and services that promote health and quality of life of the most socially vulnerable segments [7, 8]. Thus, the proposal of a resolute public intervention of the Brazilian government to intervene in this public health problem becomes an emergency [5, 7, 8].

In this light, we believe that it is opportune to deepen the theoretical discussions around the subject and to advance in proposing more consistent intervention initiatives in the control of obesity. In this sense, this study contributes to this debate by listing the main obstacles and opportunities for coping with obesity in poor women living in the historic city of Diamantina, located in the southeastern region of Brazil called Vale do Jequitinhonha, Minas Gerais. For that, we investigated the dietary practices aligned to the life context of obese women and holders of the conditional cash transfer program, Bolsa Família, of the municipality.

2. Methodology

The proposal was to carry out a single interpretive case study within the health promotion approach [9]. The choice from the perspective of health promotion relies fundamentally on valuing the context in which subjects interact socially. This perspective reflects, in part, the recognition that most health practices are oriented by social space and seeks to expand increasingly the study of socio-technical networks and spaces of social interaction to subsidize the planning, implementation and the evaluation of initiatives in the sector. Such an approach may, according to some authors, create valuable opportunities for the strengthening of current health promotion actions, especially for coping with contemporary social phenomena, including the dynamic obesity among poor women [10–12], a reflexive effort on the dynamics of female obesity in poverty from the perspective of health promotion.

In this direction, this study sought an approximation with the life context of holders of the Bolsa Família government program, from the urban and rural areas of the historic city of Diamantina, Minas Gerais, Brazil, in order to understand the dynamics that permeate the phenomenon of obesity in this group, in particular. Fieldwork totaled 24 interviews and 3 focus groups. The criteria for the selection of the group included: (1) the family registered with a local Family Health Strategy team; (2) the family registered in the Bolsa Família government program and (3) the diagnosis of obesity in at least one of its members. All these combined information allowed the selection of socially vulnerable families, using criteria beyond the purely normative dimension, incorporating elements related to the general conditions of life and well-being of families [13–15].

The instrument for data collection followed two previously established roadmaps. The first script was used to conduct the in-depth interviews—"semi-structured interview script," which contained information such as socioeconomic; consumption and food practices; work and leisure activities; and the conditional income transfer program Bolsa Família. For the focus groups, the "script of debates" was used that addressed the themes of food, the body and aspects related to the

Bolsa Família program. In the data treatment, the content analysis proposed by Bardin [16] was used. The data were compiled in five main thematic axes: (1) food routine; (2) perceptions and conceptions of body; (3) perceptions about the Bolsa Família program (PBF); (4) physical and leisure activity and (5) living conditions. In this chapter, in particular, we will address issues related to coping with obesity in the group. It is worth pointing out that in this investigation, the ethical principles contained in the Declaration of Helsinki were fulfilled [17].

3. Results and discussion

From 24 interviews conducted in the domiciles and 3 focus groups conducted in a primary health care unit, it was verified that obesity was present in women [18]. The coexistence of obesity with several chronic diseases, being the most prevalent—diabetes mellitus, hypertension, dyslipidemias and bone diseases was also observed. Regarding the age range of our research universe, age of women presented range from 14 to 56 years. In the analysis of the combined social indicators, which aimed to discriminate women subjected to conditions of social vulnerability, it was observed that low schooling was present in the group. And some women were considered to be functional illiterates. In fact, educational inequalities have been related to the occurrence of obesity in women. In general, the lower the schooling, the greater the frequency of obesity in the group [19, 20]. This profile is related to lower job opportunities, lower wages and protection [21]. Thus, the holders were inserted in occupations of work of little prestige exercising activities of day laborers, domestic workers, nannies, artisans, among others. The low qualifications of the occupations performed by these women were also reflected in low income: the average wage found was one to two monthly minimum wages.

As per family arrangements, we can characterize them as "couple with children" and "single parent" (those headed by women, without spouses and with children). According to data from the 2010 Census [22], this is one of the new trends in Brazilian family dynamics. Official statistics indicate that, in fact, there is an unequal position in the family income of single-parent households [23].

With regard to consumer goods in all households where the families were interviewed, there was a television, stove and refrigerator. The microcomputer was present in 30% of households, however, only 10% had access to the internet. Still according to PNAD, in Brazil, there are 77 million people connected to the internet. In recent years, the number of internet users has grown by 14.7% [24]. However, among the poor, the expansion seems to occur more slowly. For Tilly [15], this is one of the mechanisms for maintaining social inequalities in the daily lives of the poor within contemporary societies—"digitized," "connected" and "computerized." Low internet access in these segments limits opportunities and the majority of households did not use fixed-line telephony, but all of them used mobile telephony (cellular telephone). Mobile telephony appears to be replacing the landline telephony, according to the 2010 Census [22]. With regard to access to public services, we can now see the absence, at times the deficit of basic sanitation, garbage collection and transportation. For local health services, the biggest complaints were related to the reduced number of doctors and the enormous difficulties encountered in making appointments and examinations.

In this study, it was found that the mean number of children found was relatively similar to the results obtained in the 2010 Census [22]. Each women had, on average, 2–4 children. It has been observed that parity has been a potential predictor for the development of obesity in women, as the studies reveal [5, 20]. We also observed the presence of grandchildren under 5 years of age in these families. This profile increases the degree of dependence and fragility of these arrangements.

According to the National Survey of Household Sample—PNAD [24], the presence of children in the homes is an indicator of vulnerability in the poorer arrangements, especially those headed by women, because they have less provider in the household. Still according to PNAD [24], in this profile, there is an overrepresentation of providers by color or race—black or brown, in addition to low level of education of the reference person. Studies have shown the relationship between gender, color/race, socioeconomic position and obesity [19, 25–27]. This was the profile of the families interviewed in this study. It should also be noted that the city of Diamantina/MG has few public day care centers. For this reason, it was found that many women, especially older women, took care of the smaller grandchildren so their daughters could work. This is a very problematic issue in overcoming poverty in the city.

Regarding the leisure activities carried out by the women in these rare moments (in which they said they were "idle"), the following were mentioned: (1) manual or non-profit activities ("I'll sew, I'll weave"; "I like to sew some things like that for others and fix clothes"; "I usually take care of the flowerbeds"); (2) family with children and grandchildren ("I play with the boys"; "when I'm late I'll talk to my daughter"; "I play with my grandchildren because I like to play ball with them, I take them to walk on the court"); (3) physical rest ("I lie on the couch"; "I take a nap"; "I sleep a little"). And especially (4) watching television ("when I have a little time to watch television I like"; "I lie down and watch television"; "I'm going to watch television, watch a movie"). The frequency of watching television has been associated with obesity among women [27]. Watching television seemed be the most commonly used by the group, because it is economical, safe and available. In addition, according to Da Matta [28], everything that refers to the use, care and recovery of the body, and which as a consequence implies rest and renewal is linked to the domestic and intimate world of the house.

4. The multiple challenges to intervene in overweight in the local context

With regard to coping with obesity, it was possible to verify two fundamental questions that were recurrent in the women's testimony. Thus, for the group to intervene in overweight, it is meant following the medical guidelines. This issue reveals the incorporation of medical and media discourse operating in the group. For women, it was therefore necessary to have "discipline"; "Self-control" ("doing physical activity," "walking," "exercise," "sport," "swimming," "walking," "if you can, gym," "diet," "To do the right thing," "to close the mouth," "to control the mouth," "to stop eating," "to force") to intervene in the problem of being overweight.

For the group, facing the excess weight was still, to have greater access to health professionals (nutritionists), for them, to obtain "some recommendations"; "tips"; "guidance"; "have a follow up". In this regard, they consider it possible to control the problem. Although advances have been noted with the inclusion of nutritionists in the Family Health Support Centers (NASF) since 2008, the insertion of this professional is still insufficient. In this sense, it is necessary to increase the number of these professionals within the scope of the Unified Health System [29].

In the analysis of all the empirical material, we verified the interweaving of multiple dimensions operating in the dynamics of obesity in the group. Thus, it was possible to identify the main obstacles, as well as some possibilities to face the problem among the women interviewed. In this direction, we find that at the macro level, the historical social debt the State of Minas Gerais and the federal public power has with the Jequitinhonha/MG Valley region must be considered.

For decades, this region has presented high levels of social inequality and poverty [30]. The Vale do Jequitinhonha/MG therefore lacks a broad scope of integrated public policies to minimize the perverse effects of scarce public investments in the region [31]. Thus, inequalities in work opportunities, income, health, education, infrastructure and leisure are observed [5]. In this context of adversity, the Bolsa Família program represents an extremely positive public intervention for the families interviewed, while minimizing the effects of poverty. However, the program proved to be an insufficient public measure to transform the extremely precarious context in which these women and their families live. Poverty and social inequities in this region are therefore of a macrostructural order and it must be acknowledged that there is still a considerable gap for the local development of the Valley.

Also in the field of public interventions, we verified advances in actions directed to health and care of women with primary health care and the Reference Center for Social Assistance (CRAS). However, they need to be expanded and intensified. In this way, we consider the proposal of an articulated network of integral support for women, which includes: (1) health actions (mainly in the postpartum and puerperium periods, moments in which women signaled beyond weight gain, symptoms depressive disorders); (2) adequate provision of day-care centers and public schools; (3) psychological support and social assistance to poor families experiencing multiple conflicts, including the use of alcohol and drugs; (4) implementation of specific social programs directed to family arrangements headed by women with minor children and other dependents; (5) institutionalization of spaces for listening and dialog for the problematization of social practices; (6) a reduced working day considering the multiple social roles assumed by women that lead to stress situations [32], as measures that, in our view, are more appropriate to overcome the problem of female obesity [5].

In addition, women's social rights need to be guaranteed. In particular, the of citizenship by feeding one of the most perverse aspects of poverty in the group. Actions that promote the democratization of the means of production and consumption of food; the promotion of local food marketing and consumption directly from the producer; agroecology; the dynamization of community gardens in neighborhoods; the increased participation of women in food production and marketing through existing government initiatives, such as the Food Acquisition Program (PAA) [33], are fundamental public strategies to promote food security and nutritional security of the group [5, 34, 35]. The lack of local public actions aimed at increasing the supply and access to healthy food has been an impediment to the consumption of these items in the daily lives of Brazilians, according to a national study [36].

In our view, facing obesity in the group imposes, in this way, public actions of intervention of the State contextualized the local reality. That is, it involves broader and more integrated public measures that consider the network of interdependence that operates in the dynamics of overweight among poor women in the region. The challenge is to consider local specificities and recognize the vulnerabilities and potentialities of social contexts. It must be considered, above all, that individual choices, whether in food or leisure, are fundamentally social choices, as this study found. That is, individual choices interact with the social context and involve broader dimensions such as production, supply, access, availability, income, context, community participation and local culture. In this direction, the study carried out in a low income social context in France revealed the positive effect of a health promotion intervention on the reduction of obesity with the participation and mobilization of all local community—merchants, residents' association, users of health services health professionals and educators, public authorities and the participants themselves, who were invited to propose recreational and intervention activities. The proposal of intervention to promote a healthy lifestyle was structured in three fundamental axes:

(1) strengthening the individual; (2) strengthening the community and (3) improved living conditions at the local level and proved to be extremely successful [37].

In Brazil, intervention initiatives in these social contexts are still scarce. Although advances have been observed in the theoretical field with the publication of official documents in the perspective of health promotion [34, 35], there is an urgent need to build public initiatives in these territories. In our view, such measures are fundamental to find more feasible and decisive strategies for the success of intervention initiatives on obesity among poor women.

5. The possible possibilities of coping with obesity

In this study, we found that although some of the interviewed women were not "perceived" as obese, they "felt" the enormous discomfort from the symptoms of being overweight. For this reason, they worried excessively about the negative repercussions of obesity on their health and well-being. The external and internal social pressures suffered by obese women, especially those related to the damage to physical health, lead, some of them, to seek a weight reduction program [38]. This fact may contribute to the group's adherence to actions in primary health care. Under the SUS, the close partnership between the Family Health Teams (ESFs) and the Family Health Support Centers (NASFs) may also favor the creation of legitimate spaces for listening, reflection and questioning of social practices that are reproduced in the daily routine of the group for a better performance of the teams. The articulation along with the Bolsa Família program would allow the strengthening, expansion, consolidation and empowerment of intervention actions on obesity among poor women, promoting the universalization of care. In this aspect, it is necessary to expand the actions of nutritional and nutritional surveillance of the holders in order to carry out the diagnosis of obesity more quickly and the referral to the integral care with more efficiency. In the FHS, the creation of operating groups for obese women, dynamics and interdisciplinary support are presented as feasible strategies in the daily practice of primary health care. In this way, to refine the articulation of primary health care programs within the FHS and NASF with the Bolsa Família Program and the Health Academy Program for us seems to be a very timely initiative to control obesity in these groups, especially with the participation and the involvement of the community [37].

For the area of health promotion, intersectoral partnerships that raise the issue of obesity in poverty as a priority of government should be encouraged. The articulation of the public sector, with institutions of education, vocational training and social support, among others, can generate more favorable opportunities of intervention to the problem in the territory. More than that, partnerships can promote institutional investments in the region to revitalize the economy. The strengthening of cooperatives and residents' associations that disseminate culture, tourism, cooking and regional handicrafts is a concrete opportunity to promote socioeconomic development. Fundamentally, these actions are presented as more feasible possibilities favoring new "doors of exit of poverty" for this population [5, 34, 35].

In the urban environment, the inclusion of public spaces for culture and leisure, expansion of the retail food trade, job offer and professional qualification, income and digital inclusion would be measures with a positive impact on the control of obesity. Partnerships with local retailers to promote healthier rebates for these groups are measures that can undoubtedly favor interventions in obesity [37]. In rural areas, the state must promote agrarian reform and a secure, productive and equitable food system. That is, a model of agro-ecological family production increases access to a nutritious and quality diet in these populations. Agroecology combines traditional knowledge with technological innovations that help to address problems linked to productivity in the countryside, socially restructuring the farming community and family farming. These actions revitalize the traditional and cultural reproduction conditions of these groups in their typical forms of production and life and allow the population to settle in the interior, avoiding migratory processes commonly observed in poor populations [21]. Finally, the encouragement of research, teaching and extension projects within the theme of female obesity should be encouraged as well as the exchange of experiences in the academic and professional fields. The exchange of knowledge can be useful in recognizing successful strategies and initiatives by enriching this debate in the country.

6. Conclusion

This work allowed to understand the dynamics of social interactions that operated in the obese body profile of the poor women, from the Bolsa Família government program. And, in this way, the challenges to coping with obesity are recognized. In our view, research that proposes to incorporate relational theoretical-methodological approaches, using the perspective of health promotion, become fundamental for the proposition of intervention initiatives more resolutive. Thus, we believe that this study could stimulate new research and contribute to the debate about the subject of female obesity in poverty in Brazil.

Author details

Vanessa Alves Ferreira[1*] and Rosana Magalhães[2]

1 Department of Nutrition, UFMG/Minas Gerais, Brazil

2 Department of Social Sciences, ENSP, FIOCRUZ/Rio de Janeiro, Brazil

*Address all correspondence to: vanessa.nutr@gmail.com

References

[1] Silva DO da. O fiel da balança na história do corpo obeso em mulheres de baixa renda [Dissertação]. RJ: Escola Nacional de Saúde Pública—Fiocruz; 1997

[2] Tonial SR. Desnutrição e Obesidade: Faces da desigualdade social no acesso aos alimentos e nas representações do corpo [Tese de Doutorado]. RJ: Escola Nacional de Saúde Publica—Fiocruz; 2001

[3] Ferreira VA, Magalhães R. Obesidade e pobreza: O aparente paradoxo. Um estudo com as mulheres da Favela da Rocinha, Rio de Janeiro, Brasil. Cadernos de Saúde Pública. 2005;**21**(6):1792-1800

[4] Ferreira VA, Silva AE, Rodrigues CAA, Nunes NLA, Vigatto TC, Magalhães R. Desigualdade, pobreza e obesidade. Ciência & Saúde Coletiva. 2010;**15**(Suppl. 1):1423-1432

[5] Ferreira VA. Desigualdades sociais, pobreza e obesidade. 2014. 178 f. Tese (Doutorado em Saúde Pública) - Escola Nacional de Saúde Pública Sergio Arouca, Fundação Oswaldo Cruz, Rio de Janeiro, 2014

[6] Contreras J, Gracia M. Alimentação, Sociedade e Cultura. Rio de Janeiro: Editora Fiocruz; 2011. p. 496

[7] Minayo MC de S, Gualhano L. Estilo de vida e desigualdade em saúde. Ciência & Saúde Coletiva. 2015;**20**:4. (Rio de Janeiro abr)

[8] Kickbusch I. Na área de saúde, a abordagem dos fatores determinantes, de natureza comercial, é de importância fundamental para os países emergentes. Ciência & Saúde Coletiva. 2015;**20**(4):968-969

[9] Yin RK. Estudo de Caso: Planejamento e Métodos. Porto Alegre: Bookman; 2001

[10] Poland B, Krupa G, Mc Call D. Settings for health promotion: An analytic framework to guide intervention design and implementation. Health Promotion Practice. 2009;**10**(4):505-516

[11] Delormier T, Frohlich KL, Potvin L. Food and eating as social practice—Understanding eating patterns as social phenomena and implications for public health. Sociology of Health & Illness. 2009;**31**(2):215-228

[12] Macdonald B, Veen C, Tones K. Evidence for success in health promotion: Suggestions for improvement. Health Education Research Theory & Practice. 1996;**11**(3):367-376

[13] Sen A. Desigualdade Reexaminada. Rio de Janeiro: Editora Record; 2001

[14] Townsend P. The International Analysis of Poverty. 1st edition. Hemel Hempstead, Herts.: Harvester Wheatshef; 1993

[15] Tilly C. O acesso desigual ao conhecimento científico. Tempo Social. 2006;**18**(2):47-63

[16] Bardin L. Análise de Conteúdo. 1 ed. São Paulo: Edições; 2011. p. 70

[17] World Medical Association. Declaration of Helsinki: Recommendation guiding physicians in biomedical research involving humans subjects. JAMA. 1997;**277**:925-926

[18] WHO. Obesity: Preventing and Managing the Global Epidemic. Geneva: World Health Organization; 1997

[19] Alves RFS, Faerstein E. Desigualdade educacional na ocorrência de obesidade abdominal: Estudo Pró-Saúde. Revista de Saúde Pública. 2015;**1**:49-65

[20] Oliveira EO, Velasquez-Melendez G, Kac G. Fatores demográficos e comportamentais associados à obesidade abdominal em usuárias de centro de saúde de Belo Horizonte, Minas Gerais, Brasil. Revista de Nutrição. 2007;**20**(4):361-369

[21] Marques E. Redes Sociais, Segregação e Pobreza em São Paulo. São Paulo: UNESP; 2010

[22] IBGE. Censo 2010. Disponível: http://www.ibge.gov.br

[23] IBGE. Instituto Brasileiro de Geografia e Estatística. Pesquisa Mensal de Emprego janeiro de 2013 [acessado 05 de fevereiro de 2013]. Disponível: www.ibge.gov.br

[24] IBGE. Pesquisa Nacional de amostra Domiciliar (PNAD). Rio de Janeiro. 2011;**31**:1-135

[25] McLaren L. Socioeconomic status and obesity. Epidemiologic Reviews. 2007;**29**:29-48

[26] Sobal J. Obesity and socioeconomic status: A framework for examining relationships between physical and social variables. Medical Anthropology. 1991;**13**:231-247

[27] Poterio JA, Bernabe-Ortiz A, de MCL, Miranda JJ. Associação entre assistir televisão e obesidade em mulheres peruanas. Revista de Saúde Pública. 2012;**46**(4):610-616

[28] Da Matta R. A Casa e a Rua. Espaço, Cidadania, Mulher e Morte no Brasil. Rio de Janeiro: Rocco; 1997

[29] Rigon S do A, Schmidt ST, Bógus CM. Desafios da nutruição no sistema Único de Saúde para construção da interface entre a saúde e a segurança alimentar e nutricional. Cadernos de Saúde Pública, Rio de Janeiro. 2016;**32**(3):03-10

[30] Silveira FG, Carvalho AXY, Azzoni CR, Campolina B, Ibarra A. Dimensão, Magnitude e Localização das Populações Pobres no Brasil. Brasília: IPEA; 2007. [Texto para discussão n° 1.278]

[31] Leão Rego W, Panzini A. Vozes do Bolsa Família: Autonomia, Dinheiro e Cidadania. São Paulo: Unesp; 2013

[32] Richardson AS, Arsenault JE, Cates SC, Muth MK. Perceveid stress, unhealthy eating behaviors, anda severe obesity in low-income women. Nutrition Journal. 2015;**3**:14-122

[33] BRASIL. Programa de Aquisição de Alimentos: legislação básica. Brasília: Ministério da Agricultura, Pecuária e Abastecimento—Mapa. Companhia Nacional de Abastecimento—Conab. Diretoria de Política Agrícola e Informações—Dipai; 2010

[34] Câmara Interministerial de Segurança Alimentar e Nutricional. Estratégia Intersetorial de Prevenção e Controle da Obesidade: Recomendações para estados e municípios. Brasília, DF: CAISAN; 2014

[35] Brasil. Ministério do Desenvolvimento Social e Combate à Fome. Marco de Referência de Educação Alimentar e Nutricional Para as Políticas Públicas. Brasília, DF: MDS; Secretaria Nacional de Segurança Alimentar e Nutricional; 2012

[36] Figueira TR, Lopes ACS, Modena CM. Barreiras e fatores promotores do consumo de frutas e hortaliças entre usuários do Programa Academia da Saúde. Revista de Nutrição. 2016;**29**(1):85-95

[37] Fianu A, Bourse L, Naty N, et al. Long-term effectiveness of a lifestyle intervention for the primary prevention of type 2 diabetes in a low socio-economic community—An intervention follow-up study on Reunion Island.

In: Kaser S, editor. PLoS One 2016;**11**(1):e0146095

[38] de Almeida GAN, Loureiro SR, Santos JE. A imagem corporal de mulheres morbidamente obesas avaliada através do desenho da figura humana. Psicologia: Reflexão e Crítica. 2002;**15**(2):283-292

Chapter 8

Let Them See You Sweat: Integrating Yoga and Well-Being

Carla A. Giambrone

Abstract

Using the nested model of well-being, yoga, breath, and group classes are discussed to elucidate the physiological and psychological benefits that increase well-being in terms of health and social/environmental impact. Recent theoretical advances that detail the mechanisms at work in group yoga practice are explicated. Creating heat and release in the body are discussed regarding physical health and improved self-regulation and functioning. Recent yoga research across cultures is examined. Based on theoretical and applied research, group vinyasa yoga supports increased health and better relationships with others through increased self-regulation. Overall, practitioners across the developmental spectrum report benefits that span intra and interpersonal functioning. Additional research is needed to quantify students' change, and to delineate body type and physiology that best respond to the sweat response in order to inform dosage, acclimatization and increased well-being.

Keywords: well-being, sweat, physiology, yoga

1. Introduction

This chapter will explicate the physiological and psychological benefits of sweating, the ways in which group yoga beyond exercise and organized team sports creates bonding and community, and how, theoretically and practically, aspects of overall well-being are enhanced through group experiences of intense physical activity. The admonishment to hide our physiological discomfort when posed with adversity originates from a highly successful ad campaign by the Gillette Company to promote its antiperspirant *Dry Idea* in 1984 [2]. "Never let them see you sweat" became synonymous with success in a variety of fields as portrayed by the well-known celebrities who promoted the brand. Sweating publicly implied weakness, and has not been widely encouraged, until now. With the rise in popularity of group yoga and fitness classes, sweating in public is not only common, it is reported as pleasurable and leads to many physical benefits [4, 23]. Likewise, group experiences, specifically yoga, where demanding physical exertion is the primary activity create a sense of community and belonging that aligns with both health psychology and a biopsychosocial approach to well-being [15, 17]. How this happens is the purpose of this chapter.

2. Integrating well-being domains

A basic principle underlying the physical activity of yoga as a pathway to health promotion [7, 16, 22] is the notion that what happens in the body (physically) effects the mind, psychological processes, and overall well-being [24, 34]. Extant research is beginning to establish that there is no separation between the body, the mind, and effective functioning in all domains: physical, personal, social, and societal [31, 34]. A biopsychosocial approach is a holistic and comprehensive way to view well-being which only recently takes into account all aspects of one's life including the historical and political realities in which one lives [19]. The nested model of well-being [19] depicts four domains, or areas of a unified map conceptualized to comprehensively delineate all areas of life. Specifically, the subjective, first person domain is located at the center of four concentric circles, and is, historically, the area that has been the focus of subjective well-being research [29]. Limited in scope to an individual's reported feelings, the subjective domain (Domain 1) includes phenomenological positive or negative experiences of life.

This chapter addresses the relationship between health and functioning (Domain 2) and the environmental domains (Domain 3). The health and functioning domain includes two broad dimensions of human functioning: the biological and the psychological, whereby within the unified approach, the biological dimension functions to process genetic information, whereas the psychological dimension addresses mental behavior [19]. The psychological is understood in terms of three broad aspects of personality: temperament and traits, characteristic adaptations and identity, and adaptive potentials [19]. Whereas, the biological dimension includes the physiological functioning of the whole person. The biological context, functioning, and processes of the entire biological system are important elements of well-being that coalesce consciousness and personality [19]. The importance of the biological aspects of well-being has roots in genetic processing [19]; thus, an overview of related biological processes and physiological changes that yoga produces is addressed forthwith.

Within the nested model, the larger environmental domain (Domain 3) incorporates the social systems that people dwell and work within. Individuals are imbedded in a social environment that is comprised of networks of social relationships and social institutions [19]. The environmental domain includes the financial environment, individual's access to key resources (i.e., money, employment), and the basic state of the economy. Notably, when queried, yoga teachers in dire need of a living wage report that the social benefits of teaching and practicing are far more important to them then the financial means teaching provides [22]. Taken together, social and economic circumstances are given their appropriate weight in the unified nested model, and provide a comprehensive scope of everyday realities that impact well-being. In accordance with this model, the other domains (i.e., subjective, 1 and values and ideology, 4) are not separate as they function within and around each other. Thus, the model is nested in that preceding domains occur spatially and temporally within the domains encompassing them [19]. Integration of the health and functioning and environmental domains is achieved through group yoga in an environment of collective focus and support (**Figure 1**).

2.1 Vinyasa/flow yoga

Yoga as it is referenced here is a highly physical and challenging sequence of physical activity that involve movements (i.e., poses, asana in Sanskrit) linked with breath practiced with flow (i.e., vinyasa) connecting breath to movement, pose to pose, while maintaining deep, rhythmic breathing [4, 16, 22]. For example, one would inhale while standing and reaching both arms over head, and exhale while folding forward at the waist allowing the head and torso to lengthen over the legs. Matching the breath to the movements is the essence of vinyasa/flow yoga. Another element is drishti, meaning gaze and internal focus, which works

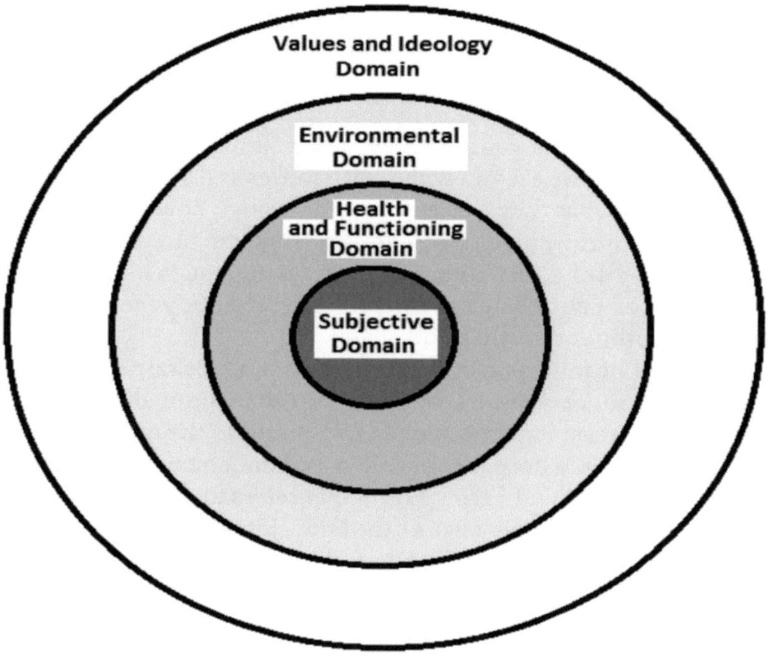

Figure 1.
Nested model of well-being [19].

to create serenity in the body by activating the parasympathetic nervous system which aids down-regulation of the sympathetic nervous system creating slower heart rate, vagal nerve activation, and lower blood pressure [15]. The potential self-regulatory mechanisms of yoga are becoming well defined in recent theoretical models [7, 15] that emphasis improvements in system-wide functioning including emotional stability through detailed self-regulatory gains [15].

Traditionally, yoga was not practiced in a physical way, but designed as an eight-limbed system of life tools for spiritual awakening [33] that include breathing practices, meditation, as well as behavioral advice on what to do (yamas) and what not to do (niyamas) in one's life. There are many informative and ever-evolving translations available that detail traditional yoga practice with origins in the Yoga Sutras of Patanjali [26, 27]. The differences between group power vinyasa/flow yoga, and group exercise classes must be emphasized. While group exercise classes are efficacious and promote health across the developmental life span, [13, 17, 21, 35] there are quantitative and qualitative differences between exercise and yoga. Foremost, exercise classes in the U.S. are typically calisthenics-based movements where individual muscle groups are activated and interval spikes in heart rate serve to improve cardiac health [32]. Conversely, yoga is a full body workout that uses every muscle group [24], and when paired with deep breathing, works to balance physiological functioning [32, 34] and assist psychological health [15]. Yoga derives from the word "yuj," which means to yoke, to unite. While exercise positively impacts the health and functioning domain of the nested well-being model, group yoga practice increases well-being by encompassing both the health and functioning and the environmental domains. Through consistent practice, with an experienced and embodied yoga teacher [20], the class as a whole may reach a feeling of common purpose by breathing together and creating a shared flow and rhythm [4, 16]. Thus, group yoga is an activity that serves to connect its practitioners to each other, and provides a sense of being part of something bigger than simply one's self [16, 22].

Physiologically and psychologically, maintaining rhythmic, deep breathing while moving deliberately and placing the body in physically demanding shapes is not easy. It requires regular practice to feel one has a sense of bodymind [31] control to stay in sync with one's breath and daily fluctuating physical condition. We all have these inconstancies, and yoga practice readily illuminates the changes day to day. How we sleep, what we eat and when, difficulties and stressors in our lives show up on the yoga mat as they are represented through how our body moves and manages the practice on any given day. This challenge can be stressful, the kind of stress that reaps benefits by persisting and overcoming, much like acclimating to heat [15], as described below. The breath is the fuel, the body the vehicle. One does not function well without the other [27].

Psychologically, one must persevere in the yoga practice rather than either leave the room literally or, more common, by checking out emotionally—daydreaming of other things. When one stays grounded and present to the moment to moment sensations yoga activates, a deeper connection and understanding of one's bodymind develops. The bodymind [31] is a term that refers to the oneness of body and mind, and an ever-present knowledge of the body, interoceptively recognized and understood holistically, not just by the mind. Through yogic movement and within the bodymind, consciousness coalesces; its activation is how perspective shifts and insights are gained [16, 34]. Through it, connection to one's self, to others, and to the wider community becomes possible [16, 22].

2.2 The purpose of heat and sweat

Sweating during yoga is both a physical response to increased and intense breathing as well as a heated space, common to power vinyasa style practice. It is also a metaphor for working hard, learning something new, and the willingness to publicly persist though challenge. Physically active over passive pursuits have been established as a predictor of increased well-being across the life-span [5, 11, 17], for practitioners and teachers alike [22]. As noted, heat can be created through focused breath work (i.e., pranayama) paired with asana (i.e., yoga poses) in conjunction with a heated practice room. However, a heated room is not necessary and should be seen as an adjunct to aid the process of sweating and muscle pliability, and at times may be contra-indicated and/or intolerable to those with certain conditions or body types [18]. There will also be practitioners who so enjoy a heated space that they come to rely on it for the kind of benefits described here. They are likely yogis who have acclimatized to the heat and achieved a level of fitness by which they can maintain their breathing rhythmically thereby experiencing a sense of ease through regulation of allostatic load [18, 30]. There is much research needed to explicate which body types fare best from a heated space, and for whom the heat remains a barrier to effective practice. Nonetheless, ujjayi pranayama, victory breath as it is known widely in vinyasa/power/flow yoga, taken through the nose serves to create an internal, cleansing heat as the exhale is slighter longer than the inhale [4, 7, 15, 24]. Moving consistently with the breath, and tolerating the increased warmth emanating through the body are necessary to feel the effects of a solid yoga practice. Thus, the essential and primary element to access sweat is heat, created and released through breath and movement (i.e., yoga poses).

Sweating serves a range of physiological purposes as it cleanses the largest organ of the body: the skin—that serves as environmental protection and helps regulate body temperature and blood pressure [8]. While rates and bodily locations of sweating vary by age and gender [18], increased internal body heat and adapting to it (i.e., heat acclimatization) can be achieved through deep breathing while moving, and enhanced through increased ambient temperature (i.e., a hot room). The regulation of body temperature (i.e., increased sweat rate, earlier onset of sweat production) during movement/exercise/yoga is critical because of the potential for lethal hyperthermia [3]. Thermoregulatory adaptations vary based on the type of heat (e.g., humid or dry heat) along with cardiovascular adjustments which result in necessary decreased central body temperature. The rate of sweating influences thermoregulation whereby if the hourly sweat rate is small, adaptation of whole body sweat rate may not occur [3]. This is significant as peripheral adaptation is a necessary component to the physiological down-regulation associated with breathing deeply (ujjayi pranayama), and moving intently (vinyasa) [3].

Tolerating heat in terms of being able to maintain a consistent breathing pattern as well as fluidity of movement pose to pose is essential in order to experience its cleansing effects. Once sufficient heat (i.e., tapas) and its release (i.e., sweating) are established, practitioners can begin to enjoy the benefits and changes that occur physiologically including increased self-regulation and improved affect [14, 15, 16]. Down regulation and sympathetic nervous system activation are often described across biopsychosocial domains as feelings of connection to others, of peace and resilience, and produces observable changes including increased flexibility and the ability to communicate more clearly without defensiveness [10, 16, 22].

2.3 Psychosocial benefits of group yoga

Implicit in the title of this chapter is the notion of being seen by others. To sweat publicly, to expose one's vulnerability in a group of potential strangers, requires courage. Recent research indicates that the ability to be vulnerable, to allow one's weaknesses and foibles to be known, is an essential aspect of living happily and whole-heartedly [6]. Why is this significant? One can feel like a fish out of water when beginning yoga—everything is different and can be slightly uncomfortable to start—the clothes are fitted, one's feet are exposed, you will need: a hair tie, a good, non-slip yoga mat, some water, a towel (for the sweat), and a flexible notion of personal space as between you and the next sweaty breather there may be just a few small inches. Group yoga classes create bonding & community [10, 16, 22] based on the human need to affiliate, to be part of a group, and to participate in enjoyable activity regardless of the inconvenience of necessary travel [1]. Similar to exercise, solo practice may support certain increased physical benefits [9], yet neither on-line nor private yoga compares to being in-person and present with others. Courage and effort are required simply to show up and be seen, and because of that investment, and risk, benefits accrue in addition to the physical and physiological effects of the yoga practice itself [6, 16].

A primary result of group-based yoga interventions is reduced stress [21] regardless of its source. Decreased stress creates an environment conducive to a sense of connection and community [5], and aligns with the environmental domain of the nested model of well-being. It is widely accepted that a positive, supportive environment increases social competence and group purpose across generations—necessary ingredients for healthy communities including the workplace [5, 12]. Improved ability to be a functional and valuable member of society is reported by yogis of all ages: school-age, to adult, to teacher participants [11, 16, 22] via increased interpersonal skills that contribute to practical and positive social consequences. For example, yoga practitioners report being more outgoing and having more respect for others due to their consistent yoga practice [16, 28]. Prosocial and community minded attitudes and behaviors are increased with yogis reflecting better judgment and caring more for others [16, 22]. Social competencies include being more easy-going, being a better communicator, and enjoying being at yoga with others. Recent yoga-based intervention research documents the positive effects of physically embodied practice to promote health and well-being [7, 10, 15, 25]. These results refer to the embodied aspect of self [10, 20], experienced through participating collectively, and the many social benefits created through movement and consistent group yoga practice [5, 7, 16].

3. Conclusions

Vigorous, breath focused, group yoga practice offers a structured, community-based way to cultivate physiological change and healing through a sense of bonding and common purpose. The group setting, the yoga practice, and especially breathing together provide the necessary tools to allow connection, personally and collectively. Being in community in this way, without added substances or dysregulated behavior, allows a purity of emotion and presence to connect each to the other, and an authentic caring for self and others to develop [10, 16]. The integration of health, functioning, and environmental aspects of the nested model provides a greater sense of well-being. For those of you who would like to have this type of experience, I recommend attending a class by an experienced Baptiste [4] certified yoga teacher who uses a hot room (between 85 and 90 degrees), and who has a healthy, active yoga practice her/himself in order to effectively provide guidance with breathing, aligned yoga movement, and pacing to acclimate to the heat.

Author details

Carla A. Giambrone
Giampro Corporation, Rochester, NY, USA

*Address all correspondence to: carlagiampro@gmail.com

References

[1] Abou-Zeid M, Ben-Akiva M. Well-being and activity-based models. Transportation. 2012;**39**:1189-1207. DOI: 10.1007/s11116-012-9387-8

[2] Ad Campaign. Available from: http://www.thisdayinquotes.com/2010/06/never-let-them-see-you-sweat-was.html [Accessed: 14 July 2018]

[3] Armstrong LE. Heat acclimatization. In: Fahey TD, editor. Thousand Oaks, CA: Encyclopedia of Sports Medicine and Science. Internet Society for Sport Science; 1998. Retrieved from: http://sportsci.org

[4] Baptiste B. Journey into Power: How to Sculpt Your Ideal Body, Free Your True Self, and Transform Your Life with Yoga. New York, NY: A Fireside Book by Simon & Schuster, Inc.; 2002

[5] Brems C. A yoga stress reduction intervention for university faculty, staff, and graduate students. International Journal of Yoga Therapy. 2015;**25**:61-77

[6] Brown B. Daring Greatly: How the Courage to Be Vulnerable Transforms the Way We Live, Love, Parent, and Lead. New York, NY: Penguin Random House; 2012. Available from: http://doi.org.gate.lib.buffalo.edu/10.1155/2012/165410

[7] Butzer B, Bury D, Telles S, Khalsa SBS. Implementing yoga within the school curriculum: A scientific rationale for improving social-emotional learning and positive student outcomes. Journal of Children's Services. 2016;**11**(1):3-24

[8] Casey G. Physiology of the skin. Nursing Standard. 2002;**16**(34):47-51

[9] Cook-Cottone CP. Dosage as a critical variable in yoga therapy research. International Journal of Yoga Therapy. 2013;**23**:11-12

[10] Cook-Cottone CP. Mindfulness and Yoga for Self-Regulation: A Primer for Mental Health Professionals. New York, NY: Springer Publishing Company; 2015

[11] Cook-Cottone CP, Giambrone C, Klein JE. Yoga for Kenyan children: Concept mapping with multidimensional scaling and hierarchical cluster analysis. International Journal of School and Educational Psychology. 2017;**6**(3):151-164

[12] Davidson RJ, McEwen BS. Social influences on neuroplasticity: Stress and interventions to promote well-being. Nature Neuroscience. 2012;**15**(5):689-695. DOI: 10.1038/nn.3093

[13] Fernández-Ozcorta EJ, Almagor BJ, Sáenz-López P. Explanatory model of psychological well-being in the university athletic complex. Proceida Social and Behavioral Sciences. 2014;**132**:255-261

[14] Field T. Yoga research review. Complementary Therapies in Clinical Practice. 2016;**24**:145-161. DOI: 10.1016/j.ctcp.2016.06.005

[15] Gard T, Noggle JJ, Park CL, Vago DR, Wilson A. Potential self-regulatory mechanisms of yoga for psychological health. Frontiers in Neuroscience. 2014;**8**:1-20

[16] Giambrone C, Cook-Cottone CP, Klein JE. The Africa yoga project and well-being: A concept map of students' perceptions. Applied Psychology. Health and Well-Being. 2018;**10**(1):149-170. DOI: 10.1111/aphw.12124

[17] Hamar B, Coberley CR, Pope JE, Rula EY. Impact of a senior fitness program on measures of physical and emotional health and functioning. Population Health Management. 2013;**16**(6):364-372. DOI: 10.1089/pop.2012.0111

[18] Havenith G, Luttikholt VGM, Vrijkotte TGM. The relative influence

of body characteristics on humid heat stress response. European Journal of Applied Physiology and Occupational Physiology. 1995;**70**:270-271. DOI: 10.1007/BF00238575

[19] Henriques G, Kleinman K, Asselin C. The nested model of well-being: A unified approach. Review of General Psychology. 2014;**18**(1):7-18. Retrieved from: https://www.ncbi.nlm.nih.gov/pubmed/29498237. (Reprinted with permission)

[20] Herbert BM, Pollatos O. The body in the mind: On the relationship between interoception and embodiment. Topics in Cognitive Science. 2012;**4**:692-704

[21] Kiecolt JK, Christian L, Preston H, Houts CR, Malarkey WB, Emery CF, et al. Stress, inflammation, and yoga practice. Psychosomatic Medicine. 2010;**72**:113-121. DOI: 10.1097/psy.0b013e3181cb9377

[22] Klein J, Cook-Cottone CP, Giambrone C. The Africa yoga project: A participant-driven concept map of Kenyan teachers' reported experiences. International Journal of Yoga Therapy. 2015;**25**:113-126

[23] Livingston R. Medical risks and benefits of the sweat lodge. Journal of Alternative and Complementary Medicine. 2010;**16**(6):617-619. DOI: 10.1089/acm.2008.0381

[24] McCall T. Yoga as Medicine: The Yogic Prescription for Health and Healing a Yoga Journal Book. New York, NY: Bantam Books; 2007

[25] Park CL, Groessl E, Maiya M, Sarkin A, Eisen SV, Riley K, et al. Comparison groups in yoga research: A systematic review and critical evaluation of the literature. Contemporary Therapies in Medicine. 2014;**22**:920-929

[26] Prabhavananda S, Isherwood C. How to Know God: The Yoga Aphorisms of Patanjali. Hollywood, CA: Vedanta Press; 2007

[27] Roach GS, McNally C. The Essential Yoga Sutras: Ancient Wisdom for Your Yoga. New York, NY: Three Leaves Press, Doubleday; 2005

[28] Ross A, Bevans M, Friedmann E, Williams L, Thomas S. I am a nice person when I do yoga. Journal of Holistic Nursing. 2012;**32**(2):66-77

[29] Ryff CD. Psychological well-being revisited: Advances in the science and practice of eudaimonia. Psychotherapy and Psychosomatics. 2014;**83**:10-28

[30] Schmalzl L, Powers C, Blom EH. Neurophysiological and neurocognitive mechanisms underlying the effects of yoga-based practices: Toward a comprehensive theoretical framework. Frontiers in Human Neuroscience. 2015;**9**:1-19

[31] Shaner DE. The bodymind experience in Dōgen's "Shōbōgenzō": A phenomenological perspective. Philosophy East and West. 1985;**35**(1):17-35. DOI: 10.2307/1398679

[32] Shiraev T, Barclay G. Evidenced based exercise: Clinical benefits of high intensity interval training. Australian Family Physician. 2012;**41**(12):960-962

[33] Singleton M. Yoga Body: The Origins of Modern Posture Practice. New York, NY: Oxford University Press; 2010

[34] Van der Kolk BA. The Body Keeps the Score. New York, NY: Viking; 2014

[35] Williams T, Guerin E, Fortier M. Conflict between women's physically active and passive leisure pursuits: The role of self-determination and influences on well-being. Applied Psychology. Health and Well-Being. 2014;**6**(2):151-172. DOI: 10.1111/aphw.12022